Th

The BASICS *of* FENG SHUI

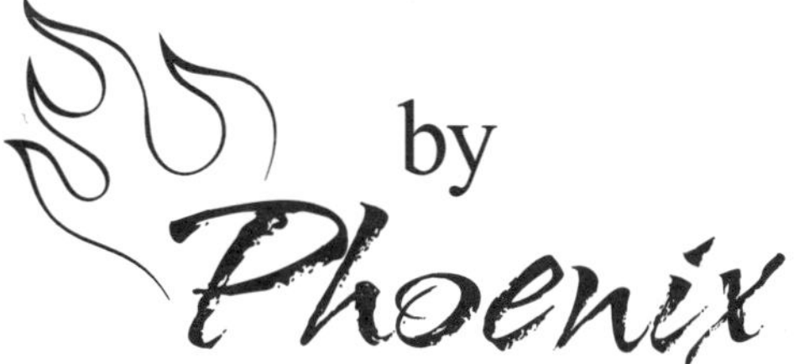

Copyright (c) 2000 Perfect Harmony, Inc.

All Rights Reserved. No part of this book may be reproduced or distributed in any form or by any means without the prior permission of the author or Perfect Harmony, Inc.

For information address:

Perfect Harmony, Inc.

2533 N. Carson St. P316 Carson City, NV. 89706

First Printing July 2002

Library of Congress Catalog Control # 2002108698

ISBN 0-9721364-0-1

Concepts presented in this book derive from Tibetan Black Hat and traditional Chinese Feng Shui. They are not to be understood as directions, recommendations, or prescriptions of any kind. Nor does the author or Perfect Harmony, Inc. make any claim to do more than provide information and report this lore.

Acknowledgments

I wish to thank the teachers whom I have had the great fortune to meet and who helped guide me on my path. One of the many things I learned is that the mark of a great teacher is the egoless ability to guide their students to become greater than they are.

To all my students who proved to me that sometimes "the student becomes the teacher and the teacher becomes the student," making me wonder if some of them were past masters who came back to make sure that I was "doing it right."

To all the people formerly of On The Scene Magazine in Albuquerque, NM who gave me the opportunity to write an ongoing monthly article on Feng Shui which created the foundation of the business I started there and this book.

To Gary and Diane Dunham, formerly of ETC Publishing House, who helped me self-publish the booklet Feng Shui Basics: Make Your Home *Your* Home in 1997 and who encouraged me to find the time to complete this book.

To Ann Wolf and Alix Seldon. Two great students of many great students, who I used in a few of the examples in this book.

To Michael "Prof. Pixel" Anderson, a great friend and very good chess player, who helped me tremendously in setting up this book. Mike's knowledge of computer programs, graphics, and fonts, and his creative mastery of them, made it possible! The majority of the illustrations in this book were created and laid out by him.

I would like to extend my appreciation to those who took the time to help me by proofreading the "preliminary copy" and the "preliminary, preliminary copy": Lynne Rathjen, Helene Minot, Katherine Starr, Lauren Stobie-Cummings, Red Wolfenbarger, Kim Monti, Deborah Anne Greco, Amanda Smith, and Amy Canadee.

To all the friends who helped keep my Virgo perfectionist side from coming out by telling me: "You don't need a preliminary, preliminary, preliminary, preliminary copy! Just do it!"

Special Thanks To

Karen "Willow" Apodaca, Linda McCarron, Robin Gile, Gary and Diane Dunham, Rebecca "Sis" Cassidy, My Mom, Amy Canadee, Bob and Beverly "The Ex" Jones, Josie "Cuz" Guido, Frankie and Nancy Sue Bartlett, Steve and Joyce Thacker, Phillip Burton, Michael "Professor Pixel" Anderson, George Webb, Rodger McCormick, Amanda Smith, John "My Bro" Tomblyn, Dean Otto, Bruce and Deana Kefover, Sue Smith, Leann Norman, Sue Sprouse, George Carver, Dr. William Downer, Genevieve Grimmett, and many, many others who helped me and believed in me during a trying time in my life. Some of you from years ago and some not long before this book became completed.

There are no words to express the deepest feelings of gratitude and appreciation that is in my heart for you. You knew deep inside you who I really am and would not allow that knowledge to be shaken by outer circumstances or other people. You felt, and in this knowing, did not and could not judge. Some of you are family and some I am honored to call friends but you are all much, much more! I hope that you would never need help in the same way or for the same reasons I did, but you can always count on me and, as always,

I Love You All

This book is lovingly dedicated to

My children: Drew, Danyelle and Dyanna

I love and care about you more than my own life! I have endured much for you and would endure more without hesitation or mental reservation!

Table of Contents

Introduction

Yes, *another* Feng Shui book! The popularity of Feng Shui at this time and the number of books written about it is amazing to me considering that I could probably count on both hands the number of books available in the U. S. on Feng Shui when I began studying it over 15 years ago.

Over that 15 year period, I have been expanding, building, and refining on the foundation which was gifted to me by many teachers. Through experimentation with newer concepts and some of my own ideas, I have created a kind of conglomerate of what has worked for me, my clients, and my students. My Mineral Empowerment Feng Shui is unique and is a very powerful enhancement in balancing the energy in your environment and in manifesting what you wish to attract into your life.

I wrote this book to help others become self-empowered. I desperately tried to keep the format easy to understand so that people who read it can do some things on their own to help bring balance and harmony into their lives.

Feng Shui is a very powerful resource and aid to what I call "being and becoming," and in returning you and yours to happiness, peace, and centeredness. This has been known for thousands of years in China and is becoming known by everyone throughout the world today.

This book is not meant to give you a Ph.D. in Feng Shui. It is the basics; the foundation of what you can learn about energy, about yourself, and how each of us are connected to our surroundings, our environment, and the "All That Is."

This connection you have with everyone and everything means that everything you say, everything you think, and everything you do creates a cause for which there will be an effect. This is a major part of how and why Feng Shui works. For example, if you want to use Feng Shui to help you sell your home, the very action of placing an enhancement, like a quartz crystal cluster, in the correct "life area" is sending a cause energy out to the Universe for which there will be an effect that can help you sell your home. If a day later, you are talking to a friend and you say something like: "I'm not really sure I want to sell my home because I put so much money into it to make it the way I wanted it to be." Now you are sending a new cause energy out to the Universe for which there will be an effect which will not be helpful in selling your home. This is very important to keep in mind as you read the book and learn about what enhancements to use in the appropriate place to bring about desired changes in your life as you do not want to send out mixed messages to the Universe. For this and many other reasons, I end this introduction by saying:

I highly recommend that you read the book in its entirety first to understand and absorb the concepts, then go back through and try some of the enhancements a little at a time so that you can feel the shifts in energy and know what works for you.

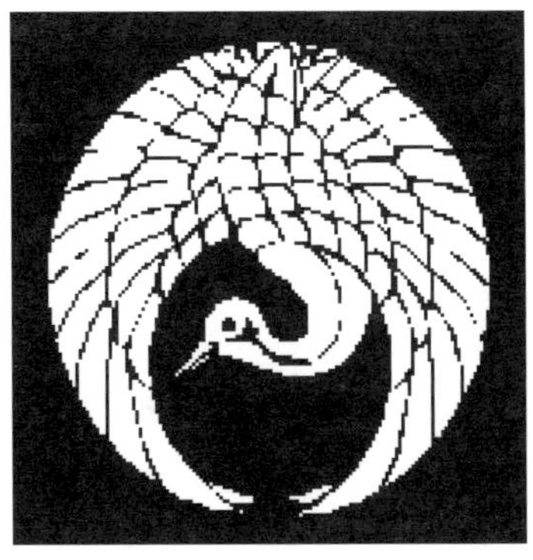

Chapter 1

What Is Feng Shui?

What if you could bring into your home or business a power that would enhance your health, happiness, love relationships, career and money flow, along with other areas of your life? Now, what if I told you that this unlimited power is everywhere, and all you have to do is "invite" it in? You would probably expect the next line to be, "for more information on this 'new discovery,' just call 1-800-GOTCHA, where our helpful operators are standing by!" (Have you ever wondered if these operators are allowed to sit?)

Actually, this is not a "new discovery." The Chinese have been practicing it for thousands of years. It is called Feng Shui (pronounced Fung Shway), which translated means "wind and water." Many concepts that today are considered "new age," are actually concepts that are "old age" which have been rediscovered.

Feng Shui is the art and science used to invite the life force the Chinese call Ch'i (pronounced Chee) into your home or business, and cause it to circulate in every room, enhancing all of the "life areas" of your environment, thus improving your life, health and destiny.

The best explanation of Ch'i, is that it is believed to be the underlying life force of everything in the universe. This life force, when it merges into our physical world, becomes the vital, bio-electric, life-giving force of the body. The closest translation of Ch'i is "vital breath."

There are many ways to circulate Ch'i throughout your environment, depending on the layout and/or decor of your home or business. I will present several methods in the upcoming chapters.

Pictured on the front cover of this book is the eight-sided Ba-Gua, a "map" to help determine where the "life areas" are in any room and/or in any structure. "Life areas" are the physical locations of sections of a room or structure which affect different areas of your life. The nine "life areas" are: CAREER, KNOWLEDGE/SELF-KNOWLEDGE, FAMILY/ANCESTORS, WEALTH, FAME/REPUTATION, LOVE/RELATIONSHIPS/

MARRIAGE, CHILDREN/CREATIVITY, BENEFACTORS/ FRIENDS/HELPFUL PEOPLE/TRAVEL, and HEALTH.

There are three major schools of Feng Shui: Form School, Compass School, and Tibetan Buddhist Black Hat or Black Sect School. Some of the schools have a slightly different Ba-Gua, that is used to determine where the different "life areas" are. I mention this because I have met many people who have bought a book based on Compass School concepts and a book based on Tibetan Black Hat School concepts which totally confused them as to just where the "life areas" are located. The best thing to do until you have made a thorough study of Feng Shui is to find which school feels best to you *and stay with that school.*

The art and science of Feng Shui can be compared with the healing science of acupuncture, and the martial art system of T'ai Chi, as all three have Taoism (pronounced dow-ism) as their philosophical basis. An acupuncturist heals you by utilizing methods to cause the Ch'i flow (vital life force) in your body to go back into balance. T'ai Chi, which translated means "supreme ultimate," utilizes movement and breathing to balance and expand Ch'i flow in your body. A Feng Shui consultant heals your environment by utilizing methods to cause the Ch'i to flow in, then balance, channel and expand it to all of the "life areas," especially any "life area" where you feel lack or limitation in your life.

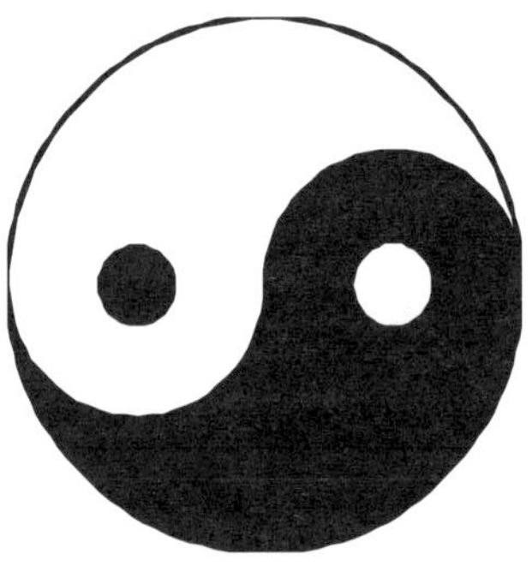

Chapter 2

Balance and Harmony

Good Feng Shui is many things, and like beauty, is in the eyes of the beholder. There are basic guidelines but very few, if any, "hard and fast" rules.

There are two reasons for this:

1. Feng Shui is very individual to each person.

2. Good Feng Shui is something that the consultant and the client "feels," especially the client.

No matter what school of Feng Shui you study, there is one constant. *Good Feng Shui balances and harmonizes the energy in an environment.* The difference between the schools of Feng Shui is in the process used to create harmony and balance. Therefore, no school of Feng Shui is wrong. They are just different schools with different techniques of accomplishing the same thing.

Good Feng Shui is based on the concept, "If you balance and harmonize the energy in your environment, you balance and harmonize the inhabitants of the environment." A dramatic example of this occurred three weeks after I had completed a consultation on a client's home. Her friend and roommate was affected by the shift to balance and started going to Gambler's Anonymous. After more than 10 years of gambling addiction, she decided in a three week period that A) - I have a problem! B) - I need to do something about this problem! and C) - Actually *doing* something about the problem.

"But isn't good Feng Shui about correcting the lacks and limitations I feel in my life?" you may ask. Yes, this is also true. Good Feng Shui can help you manifest what you want in your life, as long as it does not go against the flow of the Universe. But, you can't tell Ch'i when and how you are going to receive it. Feng Shui will balance and harmonize your life, and you may get what you *need*, rather than what you *want*.

Good Feng Shui is self-empowering, as it enables you to gain more control over your own destiny. You can't totally do away with what I call the "rising and falling", since in all things there is an ebb and flow. However, you can turn the ups and downs of life into gently rolling hills of experience rather than mountains and valleys. You arrive at a balance somewhere between the concept of "Let go and let God," but not to the extreme of feeling like a leaf in the rapids. We are all divine beings and we have the power to manifest. The main catalyst to good Feng Shui is *intent.*

Good Feng Shui is about *flow*; the flow of energy, the flow of the decor, the ease with which you can move about within and between rooms. For instance, placing a fountain in the center of a hallway is not an enhancement if you have to struggle to get around it. As we are balancing and harmonizing ourselves along with the home or business, we as individuals then gain the ability to flow like water. Therefore we can adapt to any changing situations in the same way that water adapts to the shape of whatever vessel it's poured into.

Good Feng Shui is reduction of stress. Stress is the #1 basic cause of disease and premature death. A home or business should be set up so that you have special areas to work, to meditate, to rest, to play, and to let go in. It is very important to designate the purpose of each room. You should also have no difficulty in finding anything in your space, from your scissors to the warranty on your VCR, by making sure that everything you use is put back in the same place. This will give you the ease of locating the item again. This is one reason why clutter is considered bad Feng Shui. (See Chapter 4 on Clutter.)

Does the following scenario sound familiar? You are running a little late to get to work, but you think if you drive fast enough, you can still make it to the bank first to deposit your paycheck. Where is the check??? "I thought I laid it on the coffee table! Maybe it's in with that stack of mail over there ... maybe it's in that other stack of papers over there. Oh, no! Now it's 8:55. It's in a light blue envelope—it shouldn't be that hard to find." Now you start mentally beating on yourself, which creates more stress. Something like: "How could I have been so careless!?!" You find the check and your heart rate goes down a little. You race outside to your car, but since stress creates more stress, and negativity creates more negativity, you get to your car and scream, "THE KEYS!!!" After banging around your house for 10 minutes, the whole time loudly cursing everything in the universe to eternal damnation and hellfire, a small voice in the back of your head somehow makes itself heard: "Check in the pockets of the slacks you wore yesterday."

I could add to this nightmare by having every 95 year old man and woman in town who drives under 10 m.p.h. just happen to be in front of you, but I think you get the picture.

Good Feng Shui can be something as simple as backing into your driveway at night. The better flow and stress reduction caused by just being able to drive out of your driveway in the morning, rather than backing to the end of your driveway, stopping, and then twisting your neck to be able to see in both directions of your street, can set the pace for the entire day.

Good Feng Shui can be placing a personal power symbol within sight of your front door or garage to empower you, as it would be the last thing you see before leaving for work and the first thing you see on arriving home.

Of course, good Feng Shui is making your home, *your* home. This includes filling your environment with your own energy so that the Feng Shui enhancements you have done benefit you and not the energy of the prior inhabitants of your home, apartment or business. This way you are also making it *your* space, *your* sanctuary, *your* castle (See Chapter 3). It should be a total statement of who you are and every square foot of your living space should feel good to *you*. It's the difference between thinking "I'm going back to the house." vs. "I'm going *home*." Family, friends and visitors will make comments like, "I really enjoy coming to see you" or, "I just love your place" without really being able to put their finger on why it feels so good and why they feel good when they are there.

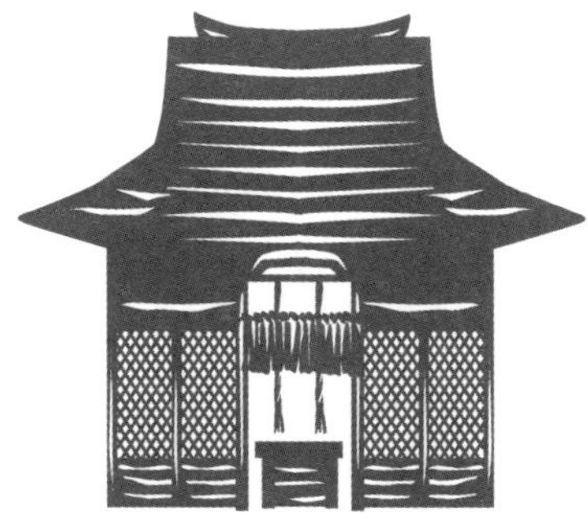

Chapter 3

Home and Business Consecration

Let's explore methods to fill your home or your business with your energy, thus making it *yours*. It is very important to consecrate your environment either before, during, or as soon as possible after you use Feng Shui enhancements.

There are as many methods to clear an environment as there are people with different spiritual traditions. You choose the way that feels best to you. Remember that Feng Shui is not a religion. It is utilizing real energy for your benefit. Magnetic energy is real. Protons, electrons and neutrons are real. Feng Shui is real. Your energy is real. We are, like everything else in the universe, made up of protons, electrons, and neutrons—positive and negative energy (Yin and Yang).

We can have someone else clear our environment to prepare it to hold our energy, or we can do the clearing ourselves. Many people will ask a minister, priest, rabbi, or other spiritual practitioner to bless their home or business. This method of house clearing is very powerful. Smudging and/or the use of incense is also excellent. Placing salt in the four corners, or completely encircling the foundation with salt, will clear the energy.

I have a favorite method which has worked well for me. It is a variation and expansion of the a traditional Tibetan Black Hat Feng Shui ritual which was first documented by Sarah Rossbach in the book "Feng Shui - The Chinese Art of Placement."

Place 9 pieces of peel from an orange in a water sprayer/atomizer and fill the sprayer with spring, purified, or blessed water. Just before the consecration, clear yourself and meditate or pray. If you are meditating, begin by saying the mantra "Om Mani Padme Hum" (pronounced OHM MAH KNEE PAD ME HUNG) out loud 9 times.

Imagine white light filling your body. Next, imagine the white light expanding from you until your entire home or business is bathed and pulsating with white light. Do this until you intuitively feel the process is complete.

Now pick up your citrus water sprayer and spray once starting at the entrance, and going clockwise, spray once in the approximate center of each "life area" in the room. Finish with the center of each room (the HEALTH "life area"). Do this in every room including a finished or unfinished basement or attic, if applicable. In hallways, just spray periodically on the floor about center and just spray once in the center of a closet or other small nonliving space. I consider a nonliving space to be any space which is just a "pass through" area, like a hallway, and any space where you would not, for instance, place an easy chair, a lamp, a bookcase, and sit down and read. I have seen walk-in closets in some of my clients homes which were bigger than my living room but it is still a nonliving area as it was not designed for anyone to spend time in other than to get the clothes you are planning to wear for the day and then leave.

Each time you finish a room, say out loud the affirmation: "At this moment I open myself and my home to receive all that is good in the universe and I will realize harmony, peace and bright blessings."

Generally, the most auspicious dates to do a consecration are the 2nd, 3rd, 12th, 21st or 23rd of any month, but *only* on a date when the moon is waxing (going from new to full).

As I mentioned in the Introduction, it is a good idea to study the Ba-Gua and read the entire book so that you can better determine what the "life areas" are and where they are located before you do an energy clearing in your home.

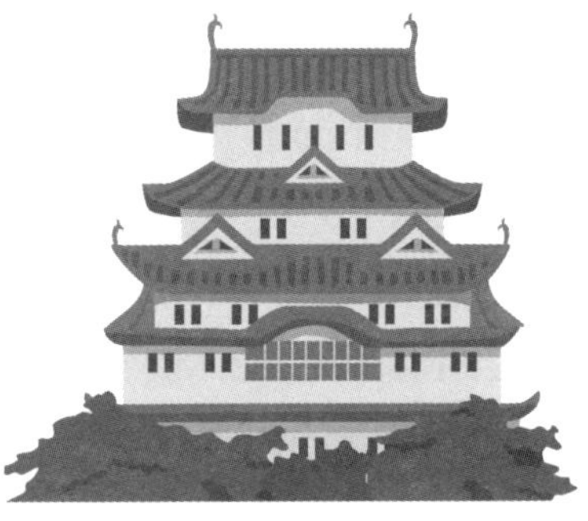

Chapter 4

Clutter

There are many positive effects of clearing "clutter" out of your environment. This clearing will also affect other areas of your life. Whether or not you believe in Feng Shui, removing the clutter out of your environment is very uplifting, on the physical, emotional, mental and spiritual levels.

My favorite story in relation to clearing clutter is: **MAKE ONE SMALL CHANGE . . . The rest will follow.**

"This is a story about a woman who did not keep a tidy house. One day, someone gave her a beautiful bouquet of roses, which she brought home and put into a vase. She placed them in her parlor. The roses, though, accentuated the fact that the vase was tarnished and dusty, so she polished the vase and then proudly set the vase of roses on the table. Now something was wrong, the table needed cleaning as well! At last, the woman stood back and admired the sparkling table and the polished vase with the beautiful roses, but, to her dismay, now the whole parlor seemed dull and murky. Before the woman even knew it, she found herself scrubbing walls, washing curtains, and opening the windows. She was letting light and air into the dark corners of the once dark parlor.

The moral being**: Make one small change in your life,** light up just one small corner, and in no time your whole life can take on a different look.

Clearing clutter may not be easy for two reasons:

1. We can easily be overwhelmed by the project to the point of never really starting, as it may seem like a Herculean task.

Your best answer is to pick one small corner to start. If you break something big down into smaller pieces, then the sum of the pieces never really seem quite as big as the whole.

2. Sometimes we hold on to things because we feel obligated to keep them, even though the item's energy may drag us down.

For example, one woman who took my classes had been hanging on to a leather jacket that her ex-husband bought for her and she had not worn in years. The energy attached to the jacket did not bring pleasant memories. She had a garage sale and it was one of the first items to go. She could not believe the wonderful sense of release she experienced!

It is important though, in the case of family keepsakes, to check with family members on items that you do not wish to retain. You might designate one or more "Caretakers" to preserve them for future generations. It may not seem important now, but it could mean a lot to others who follow you.

The best way to determine how badly we need to keep these items is by using a pretend machine I call "The Assessment Gauge". This gauge has a scale of 1 - 10. As you're clearing, consider a totally useless item (like an electric, glow-in-the-dark bowling ball) as a "0", and consider an item that is essential to your life and well-being (i.e. "to die for") as a "10". If any item does not register at least a "7", you don't need it! If you're shopping and an item doesn't register a "7", you don't need it!

I have two words for any item in your home that doesn't register a "7" - YARD SALE!

You can also consider the Salvation Army, Goodwill, etc. The point is, if any item no longer serves a purpose to you, allow it to serve someone else's purpose!

Depending on the amount of clutter, it can do anything from slowing down to totally stopping the flow of energy in your environment. This causes the inhabitants of the environment to feel a "start and stop" in their own energy flow, never really completing anything, never really coming to a firm decision about anything, etc.

There is a difference between storage and clutter. If you cannot take something out of your closet without several items falling on the floor, that's clutter, not storage. If you can hardly move around in your garage, or you can't get your car into it, that's clutter, not storage. There is a difference between things neatly arranged on a table, and so many items on a table that you can't rest your arm on it without knocking things off the table. There is a difference between nice, neat stacks of paper in file folders, and papers scattered everywhere.

Clutter in any "life area" will affect us in that area of our life. Clutter in CAREER will cause stagnation in our job or business. Clutter in KNOWLEDGE will cause mental clutter—the inability to concentrate, focus, etc. Clutter in the FAMILY area can cause blockages in our relationships with family members. Clutter in WEALTH creates a stoppage of our money flow. In other words, there is no good place for clutter other than the city dump!

In the same way that it is easy to detect where there is a negative energy flow (where things like dirt, dust, cobwebs, animal hair, etc. seem to gravitate), it is also important to check which "life area" of your home or "life area" in a room seems to be difficult to keep clean or cleared. For example, I had one client tell me, as he was pointing to the far left corner (the WEALTH "life area") of his kitchen, that "stuff always seems to pile up over there." It is interesting to note that he was constantly experiencing major ups and downs in his money situation. He clears the area, money flow gets better; the area 'junks up' and his money flow would stop just like someone turned off the faucet.

Another client told me that she always seems to struggle with keeping one room cleared in her home. She would put it in order, then two months later, it would become a disaster area again. The room is in the CHILDREN/CREATIVITY area of her home, and it is no coincidence that she was constantly experiencing an "on again, off again" relationship with her son.

You can also create clutter by overdoing the enhancements to any "life area." If you want to increase your money flow, and you put 14 fountains, 50 potted plants, change jars, and so forth, bunched up into the WEALTH "life area," the clutter caused by this action would cause the ***exact opposite reaction*** of what was intended. This is the concept of "cyclic reversal" which the Chinese call "Fu." It basically means that if anything in the universe goes too far to one extreme, the universe will send it to its exact opposite to create a balance. So, in the above example, the money flow would get worse instead of better due to the creation of clutter.

It is also very important to keep everything clean and to immediately remove any item from a "life area" that is broken, *especially* if it is a Feng Shui enhancement.

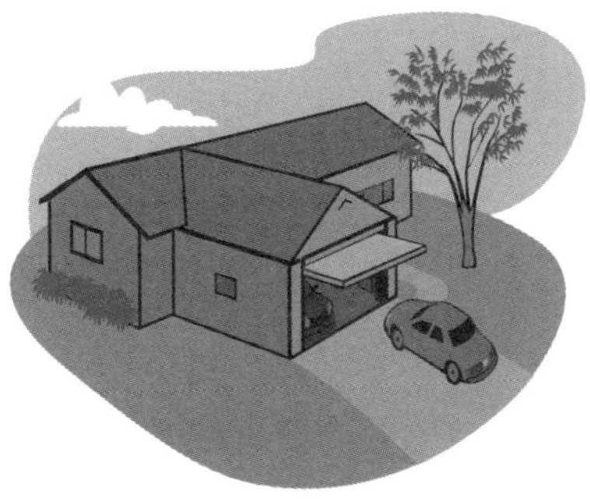

Chapter 5

Home and Business Energy Enhancement

Feng Shui "cures" such as mirrors, chimes, crystals, etc., are used to redirect and rebalance the Ch'i outside and inside the structure. They are the Acupuncture needles of the Feng Shui consultant. Let's look at the traditional "cures" used in Feng Shui.

The Nine Basic Feng Shui Cures are listed below:

1. **Bright or light-refracting objects:** mirrors, Ba-Gua mirrors, faceted Austrian crystal balls, prisms, lamps, candles, etc.
2. **Sound:** wind chimes, bells, etc.
3. **Living objects:** plants, fish, etc.
4. **Moving objects:** mobiles, fountains, windsocks, etc.
5. **Heavy objects:** stones, statues, etc.
6. **Electrical power:** stereos, TVs, Computers, etc.

7. **Bamboo flutes.**

8. **Colors:** Ba-Gua colors (see Ba-Gua map on page 126) or the full rainbow spectrum.

9. **Others:** minerals/quartz crystals, red string, pictures/paintings, folding screens, dragons, tigers, symbols, deities, etc.

Each of these "cures" has its own particular qualities and uses, and are a "cause" which can "affect" Ch'i flow in various ways. For example, sometimes a heavy object which is properly placed, such as a stone, statue, large plant, pillars, or columns, can help stabilize an unsettling situation, like holding down a job or adding stability to a marriage.

I have a theory about Ch'i flow which is important to remember when reading what follows in this chapter and all future chapters: *It is the nature of Ch'i to move in a straight line.*

The three "cures" used most often in Feng Shui are mirrors, Austrian crystals (round faceted is best) and chimes. The properties of each of these "cures" are as follows:

1) Mirrors can reflect, attract and/or bounce Ch'i. This is why a mirror placed in a direct line to your front door is the best means (depending on the layout of your entryway) of drawing Ch'i into your home. If you were invisible and looked in the mirror, what you would see is what is outside of your front door, thus drawing the "power of nature" inside.

Because it is believed that large windows are the entrance for imbalanced Ch'i, it is not good Feng Shui to hang a mirror in a direct line to a window. As mirrors can bounce Ch'i (like light), you may find that a mirror in a direct line to the foot of your bed can cause problems sleeping. If you are sensitive to energy and there is a mirror at the foot of your bed, try covering the mirror at night. One of the reasons that people don't sleep well when traveling is that almost all hotels place a TV and/or a mirror in a direct line to the foot of the bed.

2) Austrian crystals attract Ch'i to them and then disperse Ch'i in a 360 degree radius (like an omnidirectional antennae). Because it is the nature of Ch'i to move in a straight line, Austrian crystals are the best means to direct Ch'i to make a 90 degree angle into a room off of a hallway. The crystal's ability to disperse Ch'i is also why they are the best "cure" to negate a sharp corner, which is also known as a "poison arrow" (See Chapter 19 - Indoor Poison Arrows).

3) Chimes attract Ch'i to them and then hold Ch'i from continuing in a direct path unless there is another enhancement to attract the Ch'i beyond the chime. Remembering that Ch'i moves in a straight line, if your back door is in a direct line to your front door, Ch'i will come in your front door and go right out your back door. A chime is the best "cure" to place just inside at the center of your back door, as it will stop Ch'i from continuing out the back door. You should not place another chime in a direct line

outside your back door, as you have then placed another attractor to draw Ch'i out of your home. If you have a staircase in a direct line to your front door, most of the Ch'i entering your home is going upstairs. Hanging a chime between the front door and the stairs is the best "cure" for this. Chimes and bells also have the ability to break up imbalanced Ch'i.

Now that we know the properties of the three main "cures", let's use them to call Ch'i to our front door area and then bring it inside our home or business.

To call Ch'i to your front door area, hang a chime outside your front door in a direct line to the center of the door, or on the front door at center, or above the center of the front door.

To cause Ch'i to flow in, you should hang an Austrian crystal inside, in a direct line with the center of your front door, or place a mirror on the wall opposite, and in a direct line, facing your front door. This builds a canal *from* the chime which has called Ch'i to your front door/front porch area *into* your home or business (unless you have one of the situations mentioned earlier, such as your front door being in a direct line to your back door. Then you would use *another* chime to bring Ch'i into your environment.). If you use a mirror, the mirror should be large enough to reflect the entire doorway. If you stand in your doorway, and looked into the mirror, you should be able to see all of you, with no heads cut off. You should not use mirror tiles, as they give the feeling that they are dissecting your body.

To repel imbalanced Ch'i, it was traditional in China to place a representation of a tiger, fu-dog or dragon somewhere *inside* the home in clear view of the main entrance or on each side of the entrance *outside* of the home. You could use some other protective figure which you prefer or which corresponds to your decor. For example, if your decor is Southwestern, you could use a bear. In Medieval Europe, gargoyles were used to protect entrances. An angel would be an excellent protective figure.

Remember that nothing happens until you get the Ch'i into your environment. After Ch'i has been invited in using the mirror, crystal, or chime, the next goal is to cause it to circulate through every room, with more emphasis on circulating to "life areas" where you feel lack or limitation. For instance, if you feel you are having difficulty maintaining a love relationship, you need more Ch'i to circulate into the LOVE "life area". If you lack cash flow, you need more Ch'i to circulate in your WEALTH "life area."

Although I emphasize cures placed *inside* your structure, enhancements placed *outside* are also very powerful.

Many of the Nine Basic Feng Shui Cures can be used outside. Good examples would be: bird baths and bird feeders, flowering plants (especially perennials), trees, stones, outdoor statuary, bells or chimes, outdoor water fountains, and so forth.

Outside enhancements are especially powerful within "life areas" you have "squared off" (see chapter 7).

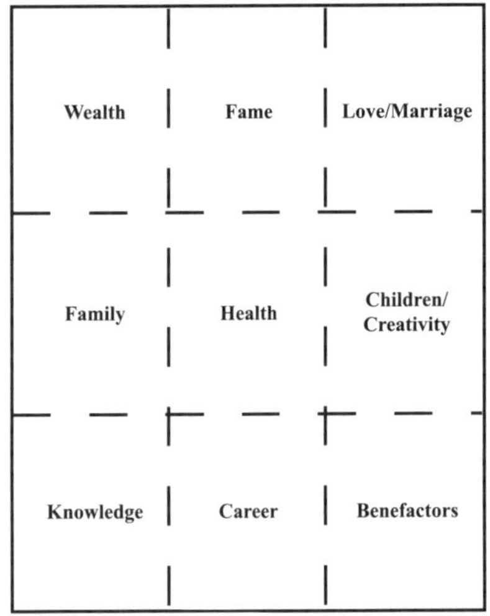

Chapter 6

Structural Ba-Gua Orientation

The Ba-Gua is just a map to determine where the "life areas" are located for the total structure, or your space within a structure, or a room . Before anything else, you must know where the "life areas" of the structure are. Remember that the Ba-Gua of the structure takes precedence over the Ba-Gua of any room.

You orient the Ba-Gua of the structure by the way you enter the front door of the structure and the relationship of the front door to the total size and shape of the structure.

If you are renting an apartment or renting a space within a building structure, you orient the Ba-Gua according to the area that is your space, not the building as a whole.

The following graphics are some examples to help you orient the Ba-Gua to your space. The arrow in each example shows the direction by which you enter the structure through the front door.

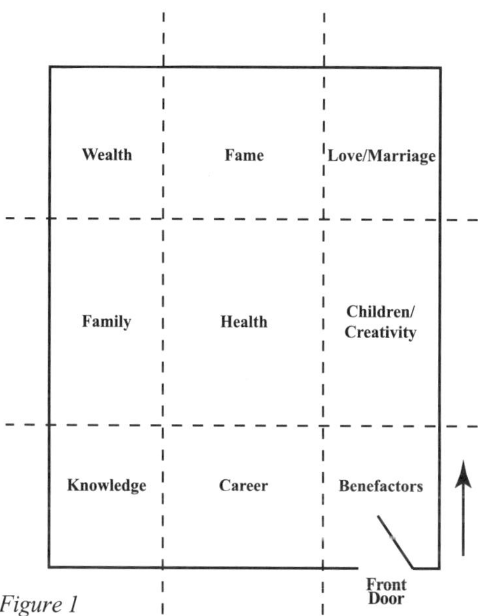

Figure 1

In this example, the front door is in BENEFACTORS of the structure and the other "life areas" are determined accordingly.

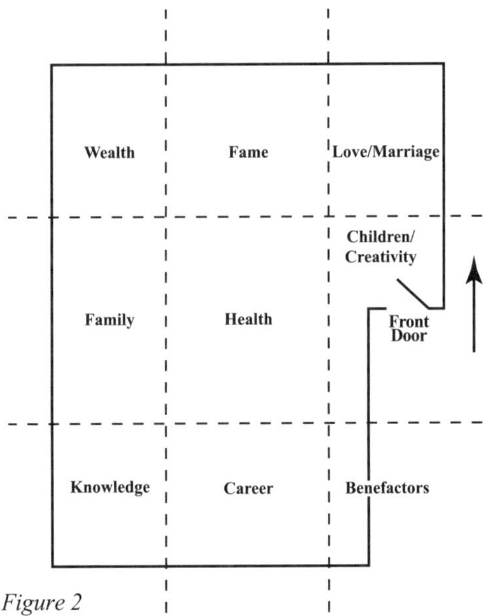

Figure 2

In this example, the front door is in the CHILDREN/ CREATIVITY "life area" of the structure and the other "life areas" are determined accordingly. As you can see, part of the CHILDREN/CREATIVITY and BENEFACTORS "life areas" of the structure are missing and the structure needs to be "squared off" (see Chapter 7 - Structural Corrections).

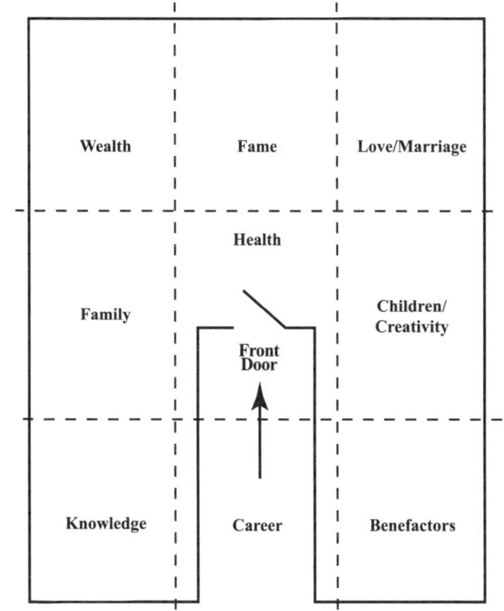

Figure 3

In this example, the front door is in the HEALTH "life area" of the structure and the other "life areas" are determined accordingly. In this example, part of the HEALTH and CAREER "life areas" of the structure are missing and need to be "squared off" (see Chapter 7 - Structural Corrections).

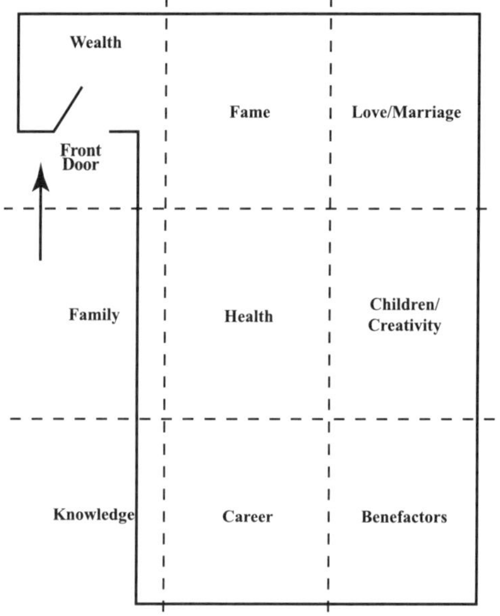

Figure 4

In this example, the front door is in the WEALTH "life area" and the other "life areas" are determined accordingly. As you can see, part of the WEALTH, FAMILY and KNOWLEDGE "life areas" of the structure are missing and need to be "squared off" (see Chapter 7 - Structural Corrections).

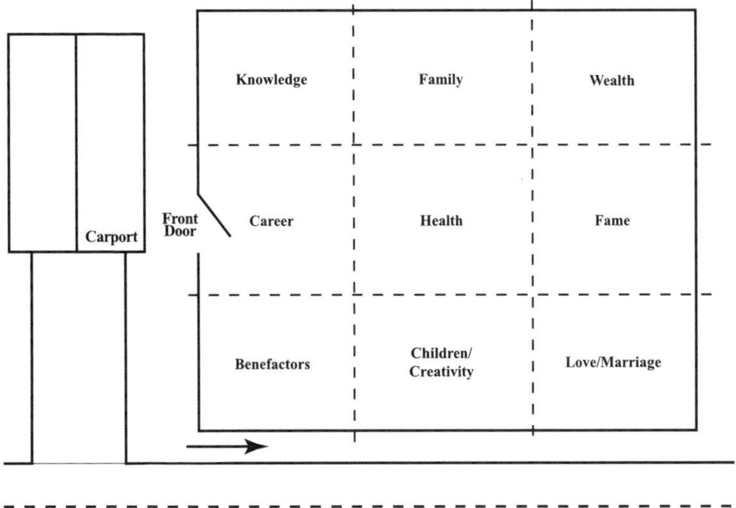

Figure 5

In this example, the front door is in the CAREER "life area" and the other "life areas" are determined accordingly. As you can see in this example, it doesn't matter where the structure is in relation to the street. The Ba-Gua is determined by the way you enter the front door.

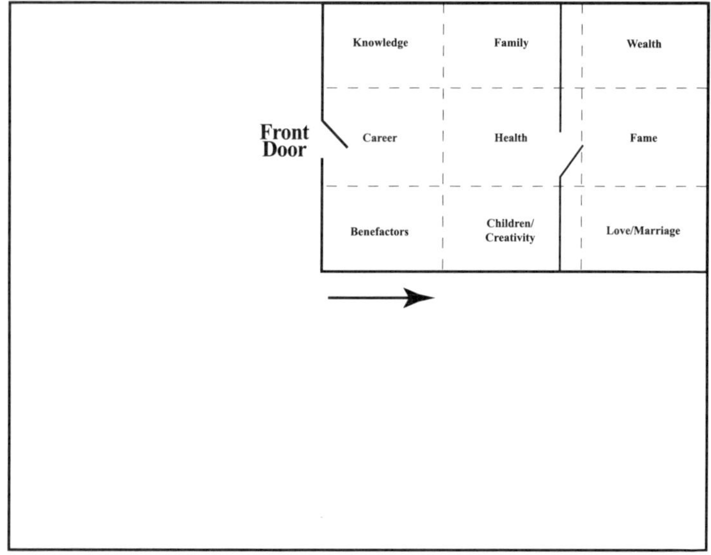

Figure 6

In this example of a simple two room office space, I wanted to illustrate the fact that if you are renting an apartment or an office space within a building; you orient the Ba-Gua according to the area that is ***your*** space and how you enter it, not how you enter the building.

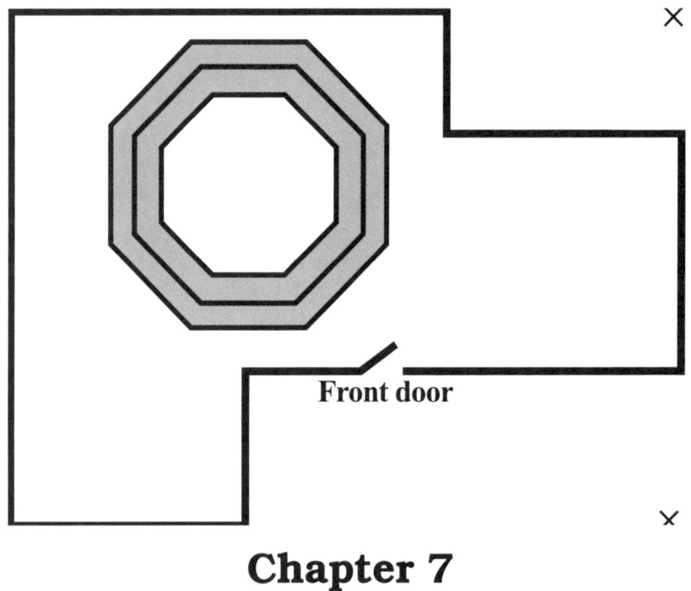

Chapter 7

Structural Corrections

We will begin our study of the process of energy enhancements which need to be done on the *outside* of your home or business structure by learning how to "square off" any missing "life areas" of the building. First we look at the Ba-Gua of the building as a whole (later, we enhance "life areas" room by room inside) because the Ba-Gua of the structure takes precedence over the Ba-gua of a room.

Looking at the structure example pictured and at the Ba-Gua on the cover of the book, we see that the structure as a whole is missing the entire CAREER and BENEFACTORS "life areas" in the lower front of the building. The structure is also missing the entire LOVE/RELATIONSHIP/MARRIAGE "life area" in the upper right rear of the building.

Not only could these missing areas cause lack or limitations for the inhabitants of this structure with their careers, love relationships and benefactors, there is also imbalance in the structure. The Chinese believe that the left side of a building is ruled by the Azure Dragon and the right side is ruled by the White Tiger. As shown in the example, the left side of the structure has more total space than the right side, causing the Azure Dragon to overpower the White Tiger, creating an imbalance in the energy. It is also very powerful to place a representation of a dragon in one of the rooms on the left side of the building and to place a representation of a tiger in one of the rooms on the right side of the building (avoid placing the tiger in the LOVE "life area").

Another reason why we would want to "square off" a building shape is that the Chinese believe that the square or rectangle is the symbol of earth and stability. The only instances where we would not want to "square off" a building would be if the building structure were in the form of a circle (which the Chinese believe is the symbol of heaven), an octagon (the symbol of the Ba-Gua), or if the building shape resembled an auspicious Chinese character or word. A few years ago, I was looking at the blueprint of a client's future home and saw that with a little modification, the structure would resemble the Chinese word for "up" (shang), which symbolizes growth and promotion, and would ensure success in almost any endeavor. Needless to say, the client liked the idea of this symbolism so the blueprint was changed accordingly.

Traditionally, the two best ways to "square off" your home or business would be to install an outside lamppost style light, or plant a tree or bush at the two points marked by an "X" in the diagram at the beginning of this chapter, to complete the shape of a square or rectangle. A "cure" of my own invention that works better is to place two single terminated quartz crystals (a quartz crystal with a point on one end and not on the other end) in the ground. Bury them about 2 - 7 inches deep and touching each other at the blunt ends as pictured below. With the points pointing to connect the corners, they create an "energy hinge" which will cause the structure to become a perfect square or rectangle.

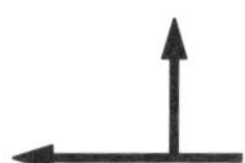

It is important that you "square off" your home or business to complete missing areas from walls that are at the farthest points which have what I call a "Heaven & Earth" connection. For example, if you have a cement slab back porch which does not have a roof over it, it has an Earth connection to the structure (touching the foundation) but no Heaven connection (nothing touching the roof or wall of the structure), so you would not need to include the porch in "squaring off" the structure. If the porch, which already has an Earth connection, *does* have a roof over it which is touching the structure (a Heaven connection), then the building should be "squared off" from the corners of the porch to include the porch as it has a "Heaven & Earth" connection. If a fireplace juts out from the structure, the building should be "squared off" from the points of the corners of the fireplace as the fireplace would have a "Heaven & Earth" connection. A wall which surrounds your home may or may not have an Earth connection (as a wall may or may not touch the foundation of the structure). But even if it does have an Earth connection, a wall would not have a Heaven connection, as a wall has no roof over it. So, you would not need to include the wall in the "squaring off."

An example of a Heaven connection with no Earth connection would be the eave of your roof. The eave is not touching anything which connects to the foundation so you would not "square off" from where the eave comes out to. You would "square off" from the wall.

As an example, the next page shows the same diagram as the one at the beginning of this chapter except I have added a *covered* porch and a fireplace. Now you would need to "square off" the home at the points marked by an "o" *rather than* the points marked by an "x" to cause the total structure to form a perfect square or rectangle.

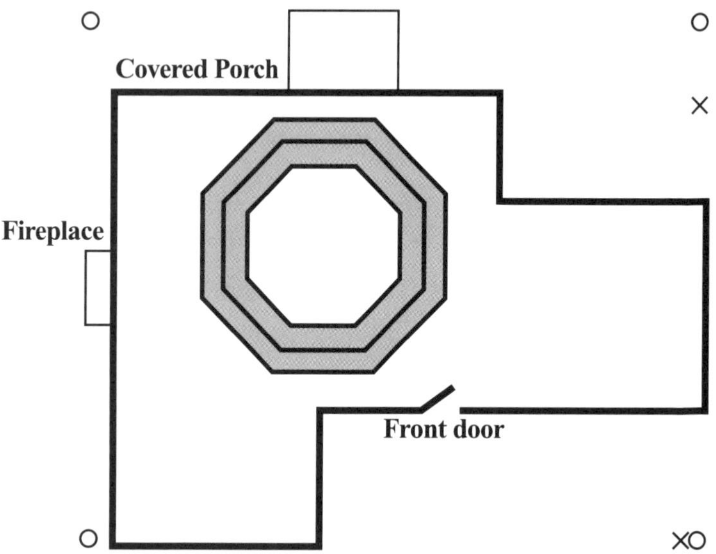

***Note**

If you have an apartment or office which is within a building structure and it is an irregular shape like the example above, it would be impossible to "square off." The best thing you can do would be to use very powerful enhancements in the "life areas" of the *rooms* which correspond to the missing "life areas" of your total space. Using the example above, you would want to really enhance the Love, Career, and Benefactors "life areas" of every room.

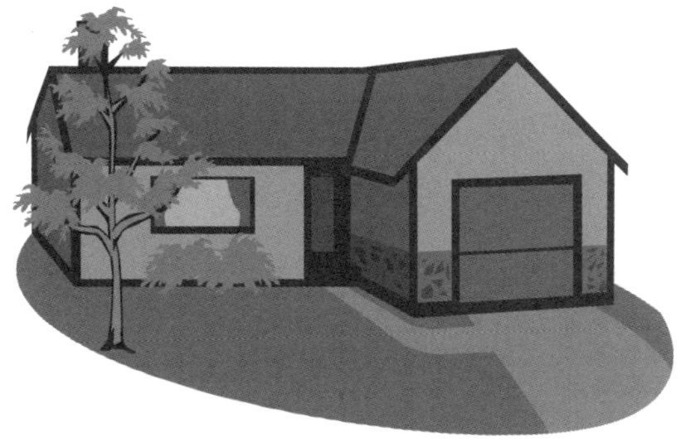

Chapter 8

The Front Door/Porch and Walkways

In this chapter, we will look at how to enhance a very special and magical place which is not in or out of your home or business. It is your front door. When you are in your doorway, you are between two worlds, as you are not really inside and you are not really outside. Many civilizations gave the same magical significance to the hearth.

Your front door, and the path/walkway leading to it, is the first impression that guests and visitors get about you and your home. This is also very important if you are trying to sell your home as it is the first thing that the prospective buyer sees.

I do want to clarify that your front door is not the sliding glass doors at the side of your house where everyone in the family goes in and out. Nor is it the back door going into your kitchen where friends always come in, and it is not the convenient entrance into your home from the garage. Your front door is ***structurally what was meant to be*** the front door. It is considered bad Feng Shui to never use the true front door. You should go in and out of it at least occasionally.

First, looking at the walkway leading to your front door, are there any "blockages" to someone along the walkway? Is there a bush or tree limbs which have grown out so far that someone would have to leave the walkway to get around it? I remember a consultation on a home where I had to walk bent over almost the entire way to the front door because tree limbs grew out over the walkway. At 6'2", I'm not exactly "vertically challenged," but regardless of one's height, there should not be anything which would cause the tense feeling of having to duck. At another home, an apple tree had grown to the point that anyone would have had to bend down and fight branches just to open the gate leading to the front door.

Second, is it unclear to a visitor just exactly where your front door is? You may need to use something like plants, railroad ties, rocks, etc., to clearly mark the way to the front door.

I did another consultation on a home where the front door was on the opposite side of the home from the driveway and garage. Next to the garage were steps leading to a deck, which spanned the entire front of the house, then you had to pass two doors which, to a visitor, could have been the front door before finally arriving at the front door. The front door was indented inward in such a way that it was not visible until you were almost on top of it. In my recommendations to the homeowner, I suggested potted plants be placed strategically along the deck to "lead" visitors to the front door. One of my Feng Shui Apprentices was with me and she recommended painting stepping stones, foot prints, or a rug-like "runner" on the deck to lead visitors and guests to the front door.

Third, is your walkway done in such a way as to make a person's steps "unsure"? As everyone's stride is a little different, the use of stepping stones or log paving blocks is not good Feng Shui if people have to use all of their focus looking down to avoid tripping or changing stride just to get to your home.

Now we will look at enhancing the front door/porch of your home. Remember that your home is an extension and a statement of you and who you are. This statement should be evident before a visitor even enters your home.

You want to note if there are any "blockages" around your front door. Are there any trees or bushes directly in front of your front door or that have grown out partially blocking it? It is believed that if you do not have a clear view looking out your front door, you will not be able to *see opportunities coming*. An example of this would be if someone asked you to display something you made at an upcoming show, which would be an opportunity to start a home-based business, but you sluff it off saying "I'll think about it." It is also not good from a protective standpoint as someone could be very close to your home without you realizing it.

Next, you should hang a wind chime in front of and above your front door in a direct line to the center of the door. This will call Ch'i to your front door *and* enhance the "life area" of your home where the front door is located. Most homes have the front door/porch in one of the three locations pictured (see diagram on next page). If your door is on the left side (see Ba-Gua), the best representation on the chime to enhance KNOWLEDGE would be (in order of best): a dragon, an angel, a dolphin, your personal "power symbol," or any nondescript chime which is black or mostly black. If your door is close to the center of the structure, the best representations to enhance CAREER would be: any water representation (seahorse, angelfish, dolphin, whale, mermaid, starfish, etc.), your personal power symbol, or any nondescript chime which is black or champagne. If your door opens on the right side of the structure, the best representations to enhance BENEFACTORS would be: a tiger, an angel, a yin/yang, your power symbol, or a nondescript chime which is black or silver.

Have you ever noticed that the higher in status that a person is, the "grander" the front door is? The doors are larger, there are columns at the front entry, there are statues of power or protection symbols on each side of the front entry like lions or pillars.

It is good Feng Shui to make your front door/porch area as "grand" as possible. This can be done as simply as having potted or hanging plants on each side of your front door. You could hang a windsock or flag on one or both sides of your front door area to make a statement and make your home or business "stand out." Having an arched trellis or arbor on your walkway leading to your front door is good Feng Shui. Having lived in the Southwest, I fell in love with ristras, especially if there is one on *each side* of the front door area. Place something on your front door like a wreath, a brass door knocker with a name plate, etc. If you feel you need more "stability" in the KNOWLEDGE, CAREER or BENEFACTORS "life areas," place large rocks, statues, large potted plants or anything "heavy" on each side of your door. They are expensive (unless you go to Arkansas or catch a sale at a rock shop), but placing a large quartz crystal cluster on each side of your door is a very powerful enhancement.

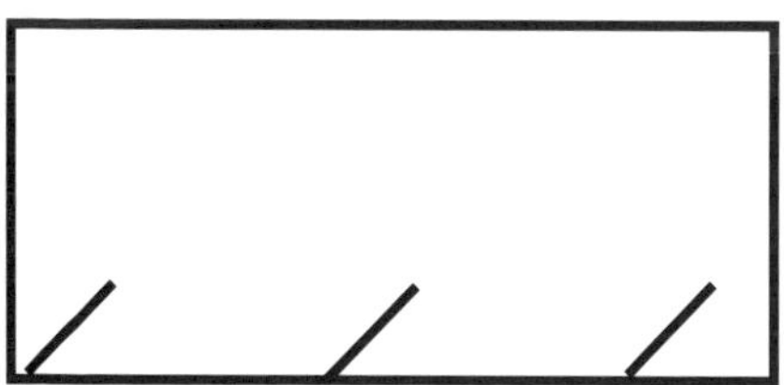

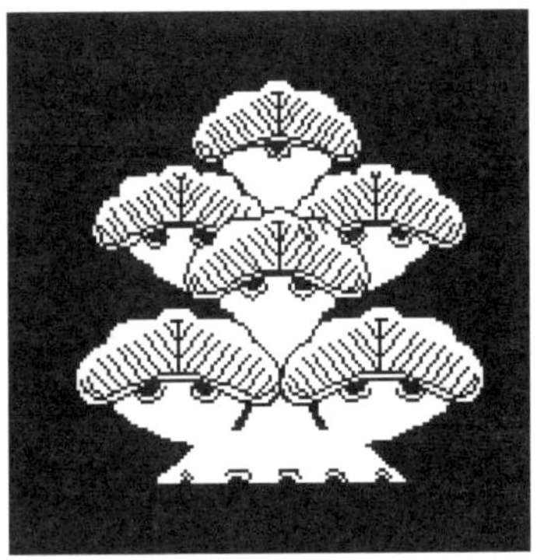

Chapter 9

Deflecting Negative Energy

Two of the most important things you are trying to achieve with Feng Shui are 1) attract positive energy and 2) deflect negative energy. In this chapter, we'll explore situations where you would need to deflect negative energy.

Five main types of negative Ch'i, according to ancient Feng Shui, are: 1) Imbalanced Ch'i, 2) Stagnant Ch'i - Ch'i which is not moving and, like water, becomes stagnant, 3) Strong Ch'i - Ch'i which is moving too fast, 4) Compressed Ch'i and 5) Trapped Ch'i - Ch'i which is moving but is trapped in a given area.

There is negative energy connected to other peoples' imbalance(s) and ill will. There is also the belief in negative entities, energies, and thought forms.

Today, we have many new sources of negative energy such as radiation, microwaves, high voltage power lines, transformers, radio towers, high decibel levels, etc.

I'll give you some examples of sources of negative energy which could be outside of a home or business so that you can walk outside around your own home or business structure and assess any problem areas.

Let's say that you walk out your front door and notice an electric pole with a transformer in a direct line to the bay window of your dinette/breakfast nook. You realize that in the three years you have lived in this home, you can count on one hand how many times you or any other member of the family have used that room. It just never felt right.

The best way to deflect this kind of negative energy is through something called a Bagua mirror. This mirror is only used for protection purposes. It is usually made of wood and is octagon shaped (like the Ba-Gua). It is painted red and green with the Eight Trigrams (the solid lines/broken lines of the I-Ching) painted in gold around the outer circumference. In the center is a small, round mirror. The power of the Bagua mirror is believed to be its ability to bounce negative energy back to its source.

In the situation described above, you would place a Bagua mirror either inside or outside the bay window, with the mirror in a direct line to the electric pole to return the negative energy to its source and deflect it from the house and the breakfast nook for the welfare and well being of the home and its inhabitants.

Let's look at another situation where the Bagua mirror could be very useful. Again, looking around outside your home or business, you notice a street which faces the left side of your home or business structure before connecting to the main street which runs parallel in front of your home/business (see diagram next page). Remember that one cause of negative energy is Strong Ch'i (Ch'i which moves too fast). In this situation, the Ch'i created by the movement of vehicles continues to flow too strongly at this side of your building structure even though the vehicles have stopped (hopefully!) before turning left or right onto the main street. The front left side of a building structure is the KNOWLEDGE/SELF-KNOWLEDGE "life area," so this strong flow of Ch'i could be weakening your ability to concentrate, focus or make decisions. It could also be causing you to feel "scattered" mentally to varying degrees depending on the amount of traffic coming from this facing street.

To deflect this negative energy, place a Bagua mirror outside in a direct line to the center of the facing street at about the headlight level of oncoming vehicles (see place marked "o" on the diagram next page). If you cannot hang the Bagua mirror on the left side of the house, drive a post in the ground and hang the mirror from the post in a direct line to the center of the facing street.

Another option in this situation would be to plant a tree to act as a buffer between the facing street and your home or business. Where the Bagua mirror would deflect the negative energy, the tree would absorb it. Of course, you would have to wait a few years for the tree to grow large enough to help.

If there is already a tree or large bush in a direct line between you and the facing street, you should be okay, but it may not be a bad idea to hang a Bagua mirror facing the street anyway. If nothing else, I'm sure your tree would appreciate it!

Bagua mirrors are very powerful. I have had numerous students and clients tell me that they successfully used one to bounce back the negative energy of a neighbor who harbored ill will against them. This caused the neighbor to either become more positive or actually move away. In any event, be very careful how you use a Bagua mirror.

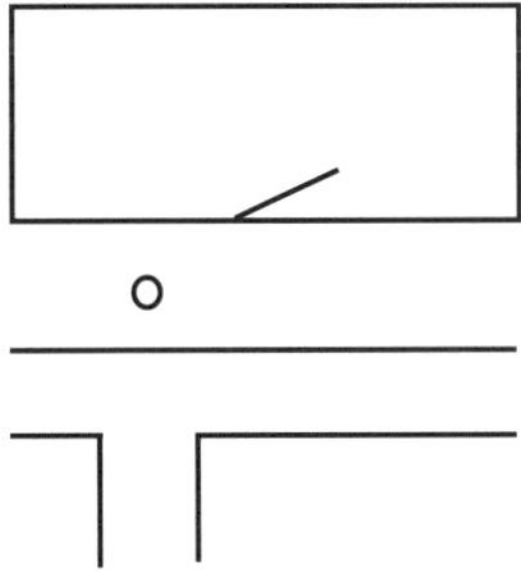

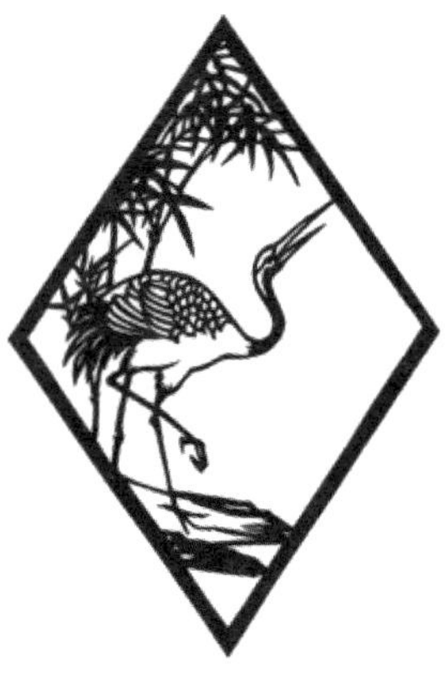

Chapter 10

Career

To use the picture of the Ba-Gua on the cover of the book or on the last page, walk into any room through the main entrance (the front door). With your back to this entrance, hold the Ba-Gua with "CAREER" closest to you. As you can see the center third of the wall area at your back is your CAREER "life area". If you have problems getting or keeping a job, or if you feel you are getting nowhere in your career, or if you want to make a career change, perhaps something is keeping the Ch'i from energizing and/or flowing to this CAREER "life area". Something may be missing and needs to be added. Perhaps something inharmonious may be there and needs to be removed or placed differently in this area.

At this point, I want to explain that the CAREER "life area" of a room, home or building would encompass 1/9 of the total area of the room or structure (see Ba-Gua on page 125). This is something to remember as you study all of the "life areas."

Looking at the Ba-Gua, you will see that the CAREER "life area" vibrates to the element of **water** (one of the five Feng Shui elements), the **ear**, and to the color **black**. Enhancements to this area could be a fountain or an aquarium (not just a fish bowl, as you want something to represent *moving* water). You might also place some coral (black coral especially, to incorporate both the water element and color), conch shells, cowrie shells, etc., in this area. Even though cowrie shell is often used to aid fertility, it makes sense to use it here, as it comes from the sea. You might consider a *black* and white Ansel Adams art print of a river on this wall, which would incorporate the element and the color. Generally, pictures should be hung in twos, or in fours in a fan shape (see diagram page 55), for greater harmony. You might place sculptures of fish, dolphins or whales in the area. In any case, be creative, have fun with it, and do what will match your decor.

Since this area also corresponds to the ear, this would be a good place for your piano, stereo, CD player, bells, chimes or singing bowls. A fountain would be excellent as it has moving water and the sound is very calming.

In the CAREER "life area" of your office, den or study, you might choose to place certificates related to your career there, or other certificates related to recognition for skills you use in your work.

I recently recommended to a client that she place a fountain on a stand in the CAREER area of her office with her business license hung on the wall above the fountain and she told me that within a week her business *doubled*.

If you want to change your career, you would place certificates in your CAREER "life area" which are related to what you want to do, not what you are currently doing. For example, I talked to a client once who was very successful in real estate but she really wanted to do more in the healing art of Reiki. I told her to remove any real estate awards or certificates which were in her CAREER area and place her Reiki certificates there.

Do not place pictures of snow or ice in the CAREER or WEALTH (see Chapter 12) areas as they would represent a stoppage or slowing down of Water energy. Ice is water that stops. There is a Nordic rune named Isa which represents standstill and translates as ice. And as the Water and Fire elements conflict, avoid any representation of fire in the CAREER area such as candles, incense burners, the sun, and so forth.

Diagram of hanging four pictures in a fan shape.

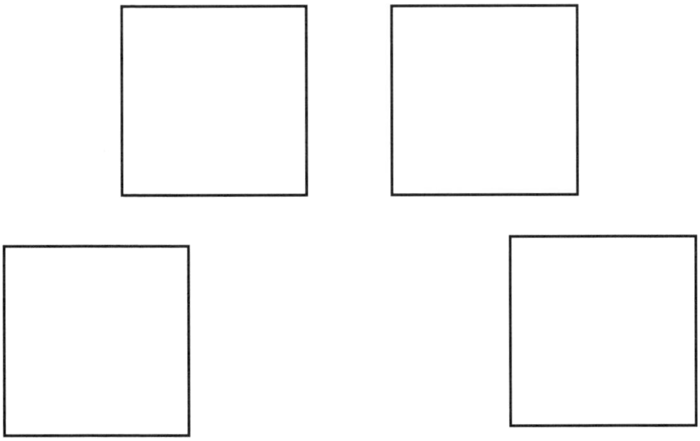

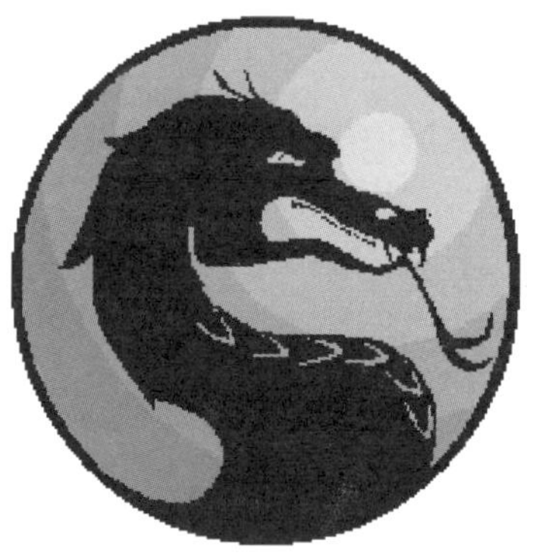

Chapter 11

Knowledge/Self-Knowledge

To find the second "life area," (going clockwise on the Ba-Gua) KNOWLEDGE/SELF-KNOWLEDGE, stand with your back to the front door entrance of any room. This area would be the near corner area to your left.

You want Ch'i to circulate to all of your "life areas," but if you are feeling lack or limitations in any particular area, then you want to attract more Ch'i to circulate in that area. For example, you may need to enhance your KNOWLEDGE/SELF-KNOWLEDGE area by drawing more Ch'i to it if you are having trouble concentrating, studying or meditating. If you are uncertain about your destiny or purpose in life. Or, if you and your spouse talk about doing something for weeks and never come to a firm, clear decision about *anything*, perhaps there is something restricting the Ch'i from energizing or flowing to this "life area."

Because the KNOWLEDGE "life area" also affects our SELF-KNOWLEDGE, it is a good idea to *always* enhance this area because, if there is something within you which keeps you from getting what you want, such as a fear of success, you will realize what is holding you back and you can release it.

"Clutter" in any area is not considered good Feng Shui, so clutter in this area can cause mental or spiritual "clutter" (See Chapter 3 for more about clutter.). Now for the bad news: almost all garages will either be located in the KNOWLEDGE "life area" or the BENEFACTORS (see Ba-Gua) "life area" of your home. If the garage is in your KNOWLEDGE "life area" and it is cluttered, the mental processes of the entire family will be hindered. If everything in the garage is stored in a neat and organized manner, everyone will stay sharp and focused.

Looking at the Ba-Gua, you can see that the KNOWLEDGE "life area" vibrates to the **hand** and to the colors **black**, **blue** and **green**. An enhancement for this area, then, could be a bookshelf—since books provide knowledge. This is also the best "life area" to have your personal altar.

To raise the Ch'i in this area, place books on the bookshelf that are *hand*-bound with either a black, blue or green binding. A "Praying Hands" statue placed in this area would also be effective, especially if it is one of these colors. You could also go with something that is "*hand* made". You could go with candles, lamps, a light, or anything which would represent "enlightenment." A favorite quote or affirmational saying that you do, or want to, live by. For example: "There is abundance for me everywhere!" would make a good wall hanging. I personally have a favorite quote by Pericles framed and hanging in my KNOWLEDGE area. You might choose to place statues or pictures of enlightened ones like Jesus, Buddha, Sai Baba, Saraswati, or angels in this area.

The above enhancements are "creative remedies," and can be used in lieu of, but preferably with, the nine basic Feng Shui remedies (see Chapter 5). Examples of using some of the nine basic Feng Shui remedies in this "life area" would be: an Austrian crystal hung in this area would represent mental "clarity" *and* draw Ch'i to the area. A fountain would represent mental "flow." A heavy object like a large potted plant, a statue, rocks, a large decorative pot, would give you more stability of your mental processes and help ground you. Placing a large amethyst cathedral-type geode in this area would be an excellent enhancement as amethyst is the most spiritual stone of many ancient civilizations and it would be considered a "heavy object." The color of amethyst is purple-violet which is considered the color of the crown chakra and ultraviolet is the highest vibrating color of the spectrum.

It is very important that the enhancements in this area go along the lines of what you are looking to enhance within yourself. For example, if you are feeling the "10,000 thoughts per second in the stratosphere" type of scattered, you would want to avoid enhancements which would be "up in the air" like mobiles, hanging plants, wind chimes, and so forth. In this situation, what would be best would be enhancements which are grounding (see above and "Heavy Objects" under the nine basic Feng Shui remedies section of Chapter 5).

As this area of the structure is ruled by the Azure Dragon (see page 39), the KNOWLEDGE/SELF-KNOWLEDGE "life area" would be the best place to have a representation of a dragon (like a painting or statue). This would not only enhance the dragon side of the structure, it would also enhance your knowledge and self-knowledge as the Chinese consider the dragon to be the epitome of wisdom.

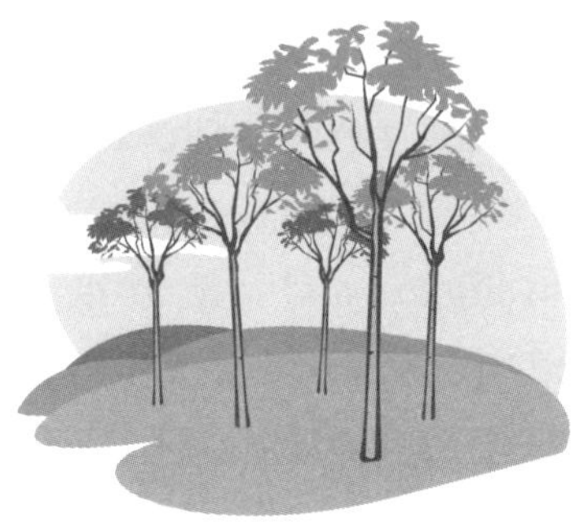

Chapter 12

Family/Ancestors

The third "life area" (moving clockwise on the Ba-Gua) is FAMILY/ANCESTORS. With your back to the front door entrance to any room, this "life area" would be the central one third area of the left wall. Some Feng Shui experts combine the HEALTH area with the FAMILY/ANCESTORS area. I believe that the HEALTH "life area" should be in the center of the Ba-Gua as FAMILY/ANCESTORS is the past, HEALTH is the physical present and CHILDREN are the future.

Looking at the Ba-Gua, you can see that the FAMILY "life area" vibrates to the element **wood**, the **foot**, and the colors **green** and **blue**.

You want more Ch'i to circulate in this area if you are experiencing problems with members of your family other than your children (which is a separate "life area"). So, if you are having trouble or fighting with your parents, grandparents, brothers or sisters, aunts or uncles, or with in-laws, then there is an obstruction, something missing, or something misplaced in this area. This is also an area you want to enhance if you have unresolved issues with a past member of the family.

You also want to enhance or check to see if something is misplaced in this area if you feel you have lost track of your "roots" or you don't feel "rooted," "grounded," or "connected."

A good example of having something "misplaced" in an area would be to have a representation of an element in a "life area" that is inharmonious to that area. Looking at the Ba-Gua, you see that the CAREER "life area" vibrates to the Water element and that the opposite wall to it is the FAME "life area" which vibrates to the element of Fire. As fire and water do not mix, you would not want to hang a painting of a lake, river, or waterfall in the FAME "life area." You would also not want to put candles, incense burners or other representations of fire in the CAREER "life area."

In the case of the FAMILY "life area," we see that it vibrates to the Wood element and that the opposite wall is the CHILDREN'S "life area" which vibrates to the Metal element.

As these two elements are considered inharmonious to each other, you should try to avoid metal in the FAMILY area.

An excellent enhancement for this area would be to place your family pictures on this wall in *wooden* frames. *Especially* a picture of the family member you are fighting with or have unresolved issues with. I know that this can be a hard thing to do, and do not do it until you are ready, but it works. No dart throwing at the picture! You want to resolve and release this so that you can go on. Place a piece of petrified wood on a stand, table, or desk in this area as it has been used traditionally as a stone to "ground and secure." It can re-secure your relationship with your family and/or release unresolved issues with a past family member by bringing everything back "down to earth" and allowing Mother Earth to recycle all of the negative energy and emotions (She's good at that!).

Since this "life area" also deals with Ancestors, it is just about the only appropriate place for representations of death, such as cow skulls, deer heads, etc. This is also the best place for dried flowers, cut flowers, and potpourri. Sorry, but a dried flower is a "dead" plant and a cut flower generally starts dying as soon as it is cut. We don't want representations of death in our WEALTH, LOVE, CAREER or any other "life area." Along the same line, the FAMILY/ANCESTORS area of the house is the best place for a bathroom, and the FAMILY/ANCESTORS area of a room is the best place for the trash or waste basket as it is going back to the Earth.

You can also go further back into your ancestry in this life area. There is nothing wrong with "honoring your roots." If you are of Scottish descent, you may want to hang your coat of arms here; or if you are of Spanish descent, you may want to hang or place a Santo on a table in this area, particularly if the Santo is carved of wood; if you are of Dutch descent you might like to place a pair of wooden (the *element*) shoes (the *foot*) on display in this area.

The FAMILY/ANCESTORS "life area" is another excellent place for a personal altar. If you go far enough back in history, you will find that *every* culture practiced ancestor worship believing that their ancestors were their angels or spiritual guides. Many cultures believe this today.

As the element of this "life area" is wood, you could choose to place potted or hanging plants here and/or hang pictures of trees, fields, meadows, forests, a house, or other buildings, even pictures of older family dwellings. This would enhance your relationships with your "blood" family, and can create or enhance a "spiritual family," as I consider this area to also represent "community."

Many of us have lost or lost contact with our blood relatives so we can enhance this area to create a very close circle of friends or peers who are of "like-mind." I have in one of my FAM-

ILY/ANCESTORS areas a painting of a forest with a pack of wolves in a circle on a mesa to enhance spiritual family. I have recommended to clients who are professionals to place certificates in this area which relate to any professional organizations to which they belong and have recommended to businesses that they take a group photo of all their employees and place the photo in this "life area."

It is interesting to note that those in the Western World are not usually very concerned with the FAMILY/ANCESTORS "life area," but the Chinese consider it to be a very important area, believing that *your* destiny is directly linked to the time, place, and manner in which your ancestors were buried. This, along with and in relation to the earth's magnetic flow, was of the utmost importance to the Feng Shui masters of old in enhancing their "client's" personal empowerment and destiny.

One example of this belief is a rumor involving the tragedy of the great martial artist and actor Bruce Lee and his son Brandon Lee. Bruce Lee was supposedly told by a Feng Shui Master that he needed to move his grandfather's burial place, as the place and manner in which his grandfather was buried would cause disaster for him and all future generations.

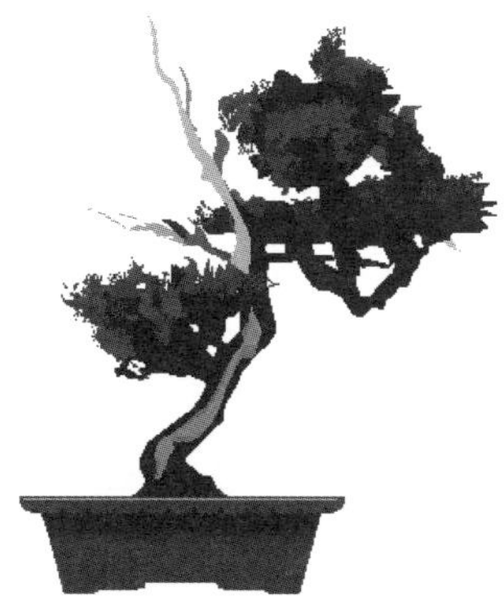

Chapter 13

Wealth

Looking at the Ba-Gua, with your back to what would be the front door entrance to any room, you see that this "life area" is located at the far left corner of your room or building. You want more Ch'i to circulate to this area if you are experiencing problems with abundance, prosperity, money or money-related matters. For example, if you feel that there is more money "outflow" than "inflow" and there never seems to be enough, then you need to take a serious look for "obstructions" or something missing or misplaced in this area.

It is also a very good idea to change your consciousness and/or intent when working with this or any other "life area." For example, guess what you are manifesting in your life if you are constantly saying "there is never enough," especially using the word *never*! A good example of changing consciousness is if you believe that "money is the root of all evil," you will always be broke, as no one wants anything "evil" around them. You have to look at money as simply an energy that is like all other energies, neither "good" nor "bad." Fire is an energy that can keep you warm and cook your food, or it can burn down your home. The fire itself is neither good nor bad, it depends on whether it is used constructively or destructively.

As you can see from the Ba-Gua, the WEALTH "life area" vibrates to the **hip** and the colors **green**, **red**, **purple**, and **blue**. I include the color **gold** in this "life area" for obvious reasons and the color **black**, as black is associated with water, and the Chinese equate water with money. Therefore, they often use fountains, aquariums and fishbowls to evoke nourishing and money-making Ch'i. Live fish, thriving in wealth-enhancing water, is considered a money enhancement. This is believed so strongly that, in China, you can buy wallpaper which has a fish scale design. However, it is very important to note that, to the Chinese, water is a double-sided coin—water that moves is a symbol of wealth, but water that does not move eventually becomes stagnant and is a symbol of death. Water which moves too swiftly is also considered bad Feng Shui. Therefore, do not simply place a fishbowl with a few goldfish in it in your wealth area—it needs to have a pump and filtration system in it to keep the water clean, and provide movement. A picture of water can also serve as a good symbol in the WEALTH "life area" as it is a representation of moving water. But, remember not to use a picture of water that moves too fast like a rapids or Niagara Falls, water that doesn't show any movement, or frozen water like a glacier or anything with ice and/or snow. Any sea shells and particularly conch shells or a fish sculpture would be more examples of good enhancements to this "life area" which represent the Water element.

Before placing water or water representations in a room, it is important to check where the WEALTH "life area" of the room is in relation to the Ba-gua of the structure (see Chapter 18) as you do not want water in the HEALTH, LOVE or FAME "life areas" of the building structure.

Another excellent enhancement is to place a plant in this area. Plants symbolize growth and fertility, and you certainly want your money to "grow." If there is not enough light in this area for a live plant to survive, silk plants are an effective substitute. A dying plant in your WEALTH area is <u>not</u> good Feng Shui. Other good enhancements in this area might be an antique teapot of silver, copper or brass. Copper, brass and silver are major Ch'i attractors and all three metals have been used for coinage, the teapot holds water, and it is used to brew something which is considered a nutrition and abundance. One client kept change in an old copper teapot for her grandchildren and it was appropriately placed in the WEALTH area of her kitchen along with a spice rack hanging on one wall which, long ago, spices were worth their weight in gold. Many kings funded explorers to search for spices. She also had several filled pasta jars on the counter (which represents abundance) in her WEALTH area. Needless to say, she didn't have a money problem. The focus of the consultation was the LOVE/ RELATIONSHIP "life area."

Wind chimes and Austrian crystals can also be used to summon positive Ch'i, and money, into your WEALTH area. Anything that would represent a "richness" to you would be excellent in this area, too. I had one client who placed her jewelry box on a stand in the WEALTH area of her bedroom. Things that you would not want to place in this area would be any Buddha's (remember, Buddha was a prince who walked away from all of his money to be poor and celibate), angels (angels know nothing and care nothing about money), or anything highly spiritual, as WEALTH deals with the physical plane.

I had one client move her St. Francis statue from the WEALTH area of her back yard to the FAME area. St. Francis was and is widely known so this was an enhancement to FAME. He was also very outspoken *against* money so he was a negative representation in WEALTH.

The above is a good example of how important it is to know the meaning and background of any representation you have in any "life area."

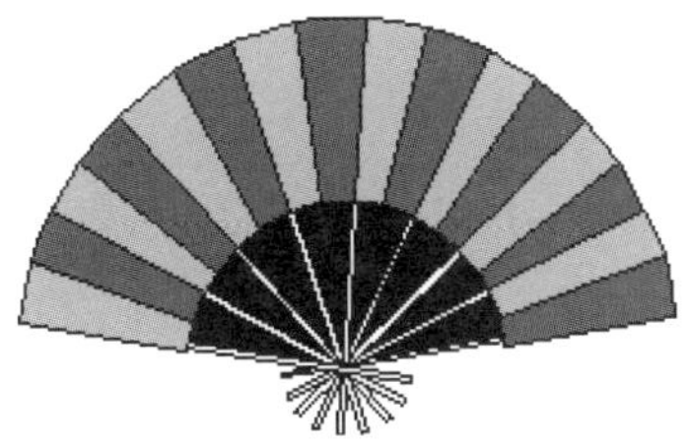

Chapter 14

Fame/Reputation

In business, it is vitally important to have a good reputation and to become "known" as one of the best in your particular market. I, personally, built up this area in my home as much, if not more, than the WEALTH "life area", as I felt that the quicker I became known and my reputation spread, everything else would follow.

If you feel that you are not seen by others in a good light or that you are always overlooked or that things you do go unnoticed, this is an area that you want to enhance.

Looking at the Ba-Gua, with your back to the entrance door of any room, you see that the FAME "life area" is the one third central wall area opposite the entrance door. This "life area" vibrates to the element **fire**, to the colors **red** and **orange**, and to the **eye**. It is very significant that the Chinese, in their wisdom, equated the FAME area with the eye, as FAME is how you *see* the world and how the world *sees* you. I also consider this a personal empowerment area, as it reflects how a person *sees* themself (self esteem and self love). Due to this, the FAME area (and the KNOWLEDGE/SELF-KNOWLEDGE "life area") is the best place for a personal empowerment symbol. A personal power symbol can be a mythical creature, like a Griffin or a Dragon; mine is a Phoenix. It can be an animal like a wolf, tiger, bear, lion, etc., it could be a saint (St. John, St. Francis), a deity (an angel), a god/ goddess (Bridget, Isis), a hero and so forth. It could be an actual symbol such as a cross, Star of David, yin/ yang sign, om sign, etc.

Enhancements, other than for self-empowerment, to this "life area," would be paintings or pictures with a lot of reds and oranges like those used in many Southwestern landscape paintings. It is important that the picture or painting *not* have a representation of water, as the FAME area's element is Fire. This is also why it is considered bad Feng Shui to have your oven next to your sink in you kitchen, as fire and water do not mix.

An excellent enhancement to this area, which was very popular some years ago in the Southwest, is to hang an "Eye of God" (Ojo De Dios) on your wall in FAME. It is especially effective if the yarn used contains a lot of reds and/or oranges, as you would be enhancing the area using both of the colors **and** the part of the body (the eye) that this area vibrates to. A picture of the Eye of Horus or the Eye of Ra would enhance this area, especially the Eye of Ra as Ra was the Egyptian sun god and the sun represents fire. Red and/or orange candles (fire) placed in this area would also be excellent, as would basically anything representing fire, such as incense burners. A representation of the sun would work well. Iron pyrite, carnelian and bloodstone are good mineral choices to place in this area. Of course, any stone or mineral such as sea shells, abalone, coral, pearl, etc. would not be good choices, as they represent water.

You do not have to go with an actual representation of the part of the body which this "life area" is ruled by (the eye) to enhance it. For example, you could place your TV in a FAME area (you listen to your stereo but you *watch* TV). Another example of enhancing the area through an indirect representation of the part of the body which rules it would be to place a telescope in this area as it enhances the eye making you more "farsighted".

You can also place an Austrian crystal, a prism, and or a light in this area as an enhancement, as light is a representation of heat (as dark is a representation of cold).

If you are working with your office, den or study, you could hang pictures, awards, or newspaper articles about you or your business, or representations of anything substantial or tangible that you would like to be most noted for.

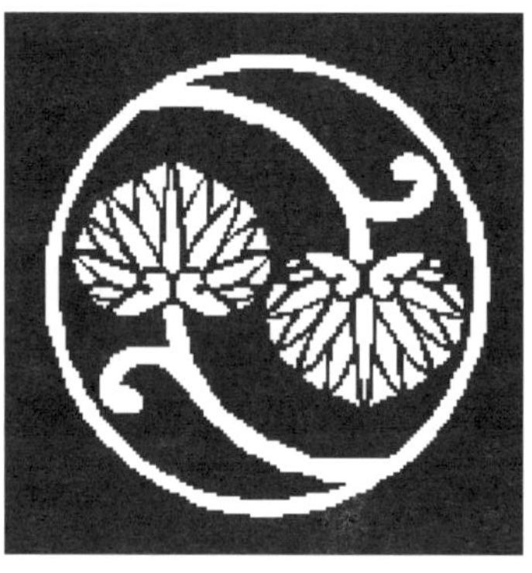

Chapter 15

Love/Relationships/Marriage

Have you ever wondered why some people are able to easily attract and maintain joyful, nurturing and loving marriages or relationships while others find it extremely difficult? Although some, due to circumstances or intent, choose to be alone, the information in this chapter may help those who are not alone by choice and feel that they do not have, or cannot seem to maintain, a happy relationship.

Although part of the problem may be due to other factors, enhancing your LOVE/RELATIONSHIP/MARRIAGE "life area" should help. Just making a conscious decision with the intent to change this area of your life for the better, while enhancing the Ch'i flow to this area, can help.

Looking at the Ba-Gua, with your back to your front door entrance, you see that the LOVE/RELATIONSHIP "life area" is the far right corner of each room and would be the far right area of your home. As you can see from the Ba-Gua, this "life area" vibrates to the **reproductive organs** and to the colors **red**, **pink** and **white**. Flowers are an excellent enhancement for this area, either real or silk, especially if they are red, pink or white, or any combination of these colors. Any kind of plant (other than cactus, mother-in-law tongues, or a plant with sharp bayonet like leaves), whether or not it is a flowering variety, symbolizes growth and fertility, which makes them a good choice for this area. The plant should be self-propagating (which represents male/female combined) and a perennial.

Any representation of birds would also be an excellent enhancement as, to the Chinese, birds symbolize the union of man and woman. The birds could be in a painting, on a fan, or even carved on a wooden box.

Once I was called on to do an energy balancing and enhancement for the home of a very happily married couple. One of the first things I noticed in their living room was a cage with two love birds that they had intuitively placed in the room's LOVE/RELATIONSHIP/MARRIAGE "life area." However, remember that the key here is *birds*. Never use a representation with a single bird on it as it would symbolize a man or woman *alone*.

This applies, of course, to all enhancements in this area (except, as mentioned earlier, plants which are self propagating as they represent the male/female aspects already combined, so you can go with just one), whether you use two hearts, two flowers, or a man and a woman in a picture, especially if it is a picture of you and your "significant other." Two hanging chimes or two bells in this area are also good enhancements. You might also hang two round, faceted Austrian crystal balls, using a red thread. Although, other than the color of the thread, a clear, faceted crystal does not directly correspond to the colors for this "life area," it does emit the full rainbow spectrum of colors.

Good stones to place in this area to bring *new* love into your life would be moonstone, garnet and/or rhodochrosite. Ruby is best if you want to enhance and maintain a good love relationship you already have.

Be careful not to place enhancements here if they also serve as reminders of a relationship that failed. Choosing angels, Buddhas or cactus is not a good idea for this area, nor anything which could represent water or a "cooling down" of the fiery love energy although a hot tub is OK. Something representing fire is very good like two red candles or having your fireplace in this area (to keep the embers burning, so to speak). Take note of the color of the candles as red is fiery passion, pink is a very sweet and tender love and white is purity and fidelity.

You might also choose a Yin/Yang symbol as it represents the male and female coming together to become one, a Sun and Moon representation as the Sun represents the male aspect and the Moon represents the female aspect.

If you are in a gay relationship or you are helping a friend with Feng Shui who is gay, you want to stay away from representations which are of the male and female aspects. It would be better to go with the placement of two hearts, two flowers, two candles, etc. A picture of two men or two women together would be used rather than the picture of a man and woman. If you are in a poly relationship, you would want symbols or pictures which would represent three or more, depending on whether you are interested in, or wanting to maintain, a triad, an extended family or a community.

Chapter 16

Children/Creativity

If you are wanting to have children or if you are having trouble with your children, such as experiencing problems communicating with them, protecting them from negative influences, and so forth. Or, if you're having a problem with your own creativity and joy, perhaps feeling that you have lost the playfulness of your inner child. Or, if you are experiencing low energy levels, this is an area that you need to enhance.

Looking at the Ba-Gua, pictured on the front cover, with your back to the front door entrance to any room, you see that the CHILDREN/CREATIVITY "life area" is the central wall to your right, which encompasses 1/3 of the total wall area and 1/9 of the total area of the room or structure. As shown on the Ba-

Gua, this "life area" vibrates to the element **metal**, the **mouth**, and the colors **silver** and **white**.

I should mention again that it is no coincidence that the opposite wall, the FAMILY/ANCESTORS "life area," vibrates to the element Wood, and the two elements are not compatible. So, if you need to enhance your CHILDREN/CREATIVITY "life area," it is important to avoid plants and anything made of wood in this area. I know it is hard to avoid wood furniture, but just make sure that the wood desk or bookcase is about 1/4 of an inch or more from the wall and the baseboard (the wood isn't touching the wall) and place something metal on the wall like a metal art object or pictures, paintings or prints in *metal* frames.

Enhancements to this "life area" would include (but certainly not be limited to) hanging metal art on this wall, or any painting that depicts playfulness to reconnect with your inner child. You might hang pictures that are fun like Walt Disney movie posters in this area. I recently visited a client's home and noted a picture of two dolphins frolicking in the ocean, which was perfectly placed in the CHILDREN/CREATIVITY area of her office.

Another excellent enhancement to this area would be to place silver candleholders on a stand, table or desk, as they would correspond to the silver color and the metal element. With white candles in the candleholders, you would be enhancing with the element and both of the colors (silver and white) that correspond to this area. Don't light the candles though as fire weakens metal and metal represents your children.

Minerals that can be used to enhance this area would be silver, moonstone, pearl or *silver thread* rutilated quartz. An excellent mineral to give to younger children is red coral as it strengthens and supports their growth. Several ancient civilizations used red coral to protect or heal their children and it was believed to have the power to eliminate negative or unbalanced energy vibrations.

Enhancing the CHILDREN/CREATIVITY "life area" will be important to you if you have to be creative in your occupation (i.e. artist, writer, etc.) or if your hobby deals in any way with creativity like sewing, needlepoint or beadwork. This is an excellent place to have your easel, desk, computer station, sewing machine or craft supplies.

To protect your children, use a Grotto with pictures of your child or children inside. A Grotto is an earthenware pot with an opening in the middle in addition to the opening at the top - it's like a niche that you can move from one place to another. I have also seen metal shrines which are like a dollhouse where you can place something inside like a picture of your child(ren) to protect them.

To reconnect with a child, find an old "Happy Mothers Day/Happy Fathers Day" card or a "birthday card" that your child hand made for you when he or she was in school and there was that special connection between you and your child. Pictures or paintings of a man or woman with a baby, depicting the bond between parent and child would also be a good enhancement to place in this area.

To increase your energy levels and/or bring out your own inner child, you could place pictures of children running or playing or pictures of animals frolicking.

If you are trying to have or adopt a child, place a cowrie shell (especially the type of cowrie known as Ovula Ovum) in this area. As all life originated from the sea, it is a powerful symbol. Other fertility symbols would be a picture or statue of a rabbit or a representation of an egg.

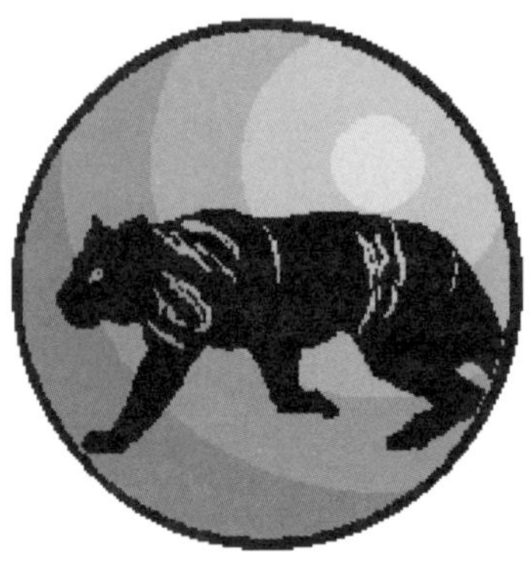

Chapter 17

Benefactors/Friends/Helpful People/Travel

The BENEFACTORS/HELPFUL PEOPLE "life area" is of great importance to everyone, especially if you are in business.

This "life area" is just as important as the WEALTH "life area". Benefactors are people, or members of our family, who help us financially when we are in need. Benefactors can also be mentors who willingly give their time, experience, and advice to help guide us in positive directions. Miyamoto Musahi, the great Japanese Samurai who wrote "The Book Of Five Rings," stated that, "The teacher is as the needle, the disciple is as thread." One should think deeply about this statement, as a great teacher or mentor should be "as the needle" to guide the student (thread) to the right answers.

Benefactors can also help us *maintain* wealth, not just accumulate it. A benefactor could be your financial planner, accountant, lawyer, or business manager. If you are buying or selling a house, a benefactor would be your real estate agent, the banker who would approve the loan, and so forth. If you are ill, a benefactor is the right health practitioner for you.

A good example of Helpful People, if you are in business, would be people who refer you to others through good "word-of-mouth." They could also be good employees who take to heart the welfare of the business.

In addition to the above, if you feel that you do not have any close friends, if you feel lonely or isolated, or if you feel that you have difficulty meeting and connecting to others, then this is an area you want to enhance. A good mineral to place in your BENEFACTORS area for this would be the form of barite known as the Desert Rose.

Looking at the Ba-Gua, with your back to the front door entrance of any room, you see that the BENEFACTORS/HELPFUL PEOPLE "life area" is the near right corner area. As shown in the Ba-Gua, this area resonates to the **head**, and the colors **white**, **gray** and **black**.

A very good enhancement for this area would be to place something here with the Yin/Yang symbol. Not only are you using two of the colors (white and black), but this symbol represents balance and harmony, which you would want in your relationships with your benefactors and friends. Another enhancement for this area would be to put a stand with a bust on it (which represents the head) of someone you admire. It would be particularly auspicious if the bust is white, gray, or black. A bust would also be one of the standard Feng Shui cures—a "heavy object," which would symbolize *stability* in your relationships with benefactors and helpful people.

When I told a client that this area vibrates to the head, he picked up his hat rack, and moved it into the BENEFACTORS area. I liked the idea especially with the many hats which were on the hat rack as this is an area where it is good to have something numerous. Another client had a painting of a forest in his BENEFACTORS area and I suggested he consider every tree to be a benefactor to him.

If you want a powerful symbol in this area, buy a stand (in white, gray, or black) that looks like a *pillar*. This would add longevity, strength and stability in these relationships, for long after ancient buildings have fallen down, the pillars will still stand for many centuries to come. Even when you have driven by a house that has burned down, you will see that the brick fireplace is still standing and will for years to come.

Placing a large quartz crystal cluster in this area is an excellent enhancement and my personal favorite. A large cluster would be considered a "heavy object" and all of the crystals grouped on the cluster would represent a lot of benefactors all grouped together for you! Minerals to place on the cluster would be magnetite (lodestone), a geode which has the colors for the area, and tourmalated quartz. As this area is the area which is ruled by the "White Tiger", BENEFACTORS would be the best "life area" to place a representation of a tiger. It would not only enhance the "tiger" side of the building (See Chapter 5), it would also give us strong, protective benefactors.

The BENEFACTORS area is the best place to have religious/spiritual representations like Jesus, Buddha, Saints, Angels, Kwan Yin, Ganesh, Rhiannon, etc. Ganesh is my favorite in the BENEFACTORS area as he is the "remover of all obstacles." I have never had anyone, that I know of who was open to using a representation of this deity, not experience a positive change after placing Ganesh in this area.

A globe or world map, posters and pictures of places you have been, or even better, places you would like to go, are also good enhancements in this area as it also relates to travel.

Pictures of close friends, mentors, or people who have helped you throughout your life is a very good enhancement for this area. I had a client who wanted to place a picture of her grandmother in her BENEFACTORS area rather than her FAMILY/ANCESTORS area as her grandmother had helped her all her life and my client felt that she was still watching over her after she passed on.

Placing gifts you have received from loving, caring friends is also very powerful in this area. On one home consultation, I saw a framed needlepoint in the clients' WEALTH area which said "Bye Mary!" I didn't want it in her WEALTH area as I didn't want her money to go bye bye. After struggling to try to think of where to place it, I asked her where she got it and she told me that over 100 of her coworkers chipped in to have it made for her as a retirement gift. This made it easy to place in her BENEFACTORS area with the energy of 100 coworkers wishing her well.

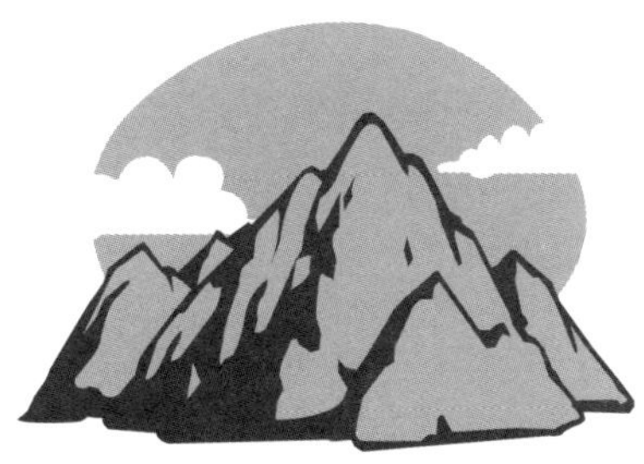

Chapter 18

Health

Now we will enhance one of the most important "life areas" of all—the HEALTH area. This area, like our physical body, is often neglected or taken for granted until something happens to make us realize how important it is to have good health. Regardless of your current state of health, *everyone* should enhance the Ch'i flow to this "life area".

I feel it is important that you understand that enhancing the HEALTH "life area" is not a *replacement* for seeking attention from a medical professional if you are currently experiencing illness, or if you experience illness in the future, but balancing the energy in this area can help.

Enhancing the BENEFACTORS "life area" can help you too, depending on the particular condition, to attract the right healing professional. A medical professional is definitely a "benefactor" to you if you are experiencing a loss of your good health, or if you want to maintain and improve your current state of good health (see Chapter 17).

Looking at the Ba-Gua, with your back to the front door entrance of any room, you see that the HEALTH "life area" is the center. It is the "heart" of the house or room and encompasses the central 1/9th of the total space of the building structure or room area. As shown in the Ba-Gua, this area resonates to the element **earth**, the color **yellow**, and the **middle body**. In Chinese medicine, the five major organs are contained in the middle body (Apparently you can live without your brain - I always have!). It is interesting to note the Ba-Gua of Chinese Medicine compared to the Ba-Gua of Feng Shui. In Chinese Medicine, the heart is red and Fire (FAME), the lungs are white and Metal (CHILDREN), the kidneys are black and Water (CAREER), the spleen is yellow and Earth (HEALTH), and the liver is green and Wood (FAMILY).

There are some Feng Shui practitioners who combine the HEALTH "life area" with the FAMILY "life area." They can probably pull out as many testimonials as I can after enhancing the HEALTH area but, for the reason stated above (the Ba-Gua of Chinese Medicine), and as I mentioned in Chapter 11, I cannot combine the two areas.

Due to the fact that the HEALTH "life area" is the center of a room, there are mainly two rooms where we can place enhancements without restricting ease of movement, with the exception of the use of throw rugs with earth tones (and at least some yellow): the living room (as the coffee table is often as close to the center as we can get) and the dining room (as the dining room table is almost always placed in the center of the dining room). Both rooms are very powerful for enhancements as, in most of the homes I've seen, the front door opens into the living room area so this is the room where the Ch'i enters first and is the strongest. The dining room, in both eastern and western tradition, is a very significant room, as it is where the family gathers to share nourishment and abundance, and it is where we serve honored guests.

An excellent enhancement for the dining room would be to place an assortment of fruit on the dining room table (the more yellow fruit you use, the better). You can really enhance this area if you place the fruit in an *earth*enware bowl. The doilies and/or placemats on your table could be yellow or earth tone colors with at least some shade(s) of yellow.

My favorite enhancement for the living room (which I have done myself), is to place a quartz crystal cluster in the center of the coffee table. The larger and heavier the cluster - the more stable your health. Then place minerals which have been known for their healing properties on the cluster (see Chapter 20 - Mineral Empowerment Feng Shui). Amber is the color of this "life area" and is the most powerful healing stone. Bloodstone (although not the exact color, it still comes from the earth) has also been used by many civilizations as a healing stone. Bone is also a good choice as, if you go far enough back in time, *every* civilization believed that if you possessed or wore the bone of a particular animal, you would take on the strength and qualities of that animal.

One idea that I came up with while struggling to enhance the center of a room, was that I didn't have to be confined to the floor, walls and furniture to do something in HEALTH, I could ***go up***! I looked up and it occurred to me that there is usually a light fixture or ceiling fan in the center of every room. Where you have a ceiling fan or lamp in the middle of your room, you can string amber stones together and hang them from the light or fan or you could use the stringed stones to lengthen the pullchain of the lamp or fan.

Other good enhancements for the HEALTH area of the living room might be a collection of health and healing books or magazines in or on the coffee table. I placed a set of Chinese Therapy Balls (also known as Harmony Balls) on my coffee table. Anything earthen (made of clay) or stone would be good too as you are using a *direct* representation of the Earth element. You can also enhance this area with candles, incense burners, or other representations of the Fire element, as the Chinese believe that

Fire creates Earth and would thus be an *indirect* element enhancement.

A representation of Kwan-Yin is most powerful in the HEALTH area. She is the Chinese goddess of healing, compassion and mercy. Her Chinese title, which translates "Born of the Lotus" signifies "she who hears all prayers."

Do not place any representations of the Water element, like a fountain or sea shells, and try to avoid the Wood element (plants) in the HEALTH area as the Chinese believe that Wood depletes Earth and Water erodes Earth. As the Earth element represents our physical bodies and our health, anything which would deplete or erode our health would not be a good thing, especially the Water element. For example, how was the Grand Canyon formed? The Colorado River ate it away! In Miami, machines are used to replenish the beaches with sand. If this had not been done for the past several years, most of the beachfront hotels would have water up to at least their 1st floor. If you give Water enough time, it will erode *anything*! I am personally not quite so rigid about plants placed in the HEALTH area which are healing. I have been in homes which had aloe vera and/or medicinal herb plants in this area and they felt very positive. And, as they symbolize strength and uprightness, bamboo plants have also felt positive to me.

In enhancing HEALTH of the building structure or home, you are looking at the 1/9 total space in the center. If you were to draw a tic-tac-toe over a floor plan of your house (see diagram in Chapter 19 and the Ba-Gua in a Square Layout on page 125), HEALTH could take in, for example, the upper part of the living room, the lower part of the kitchen, part of a hallway and part of a bathroom. To enhance HEALTH of the house, you could use earth tone throw rugs or amber hung from light fixtures/ceiling fans in one or more of these areas. In hallways, you could hang pictures which represent Earth, like pictures of mountains, which would also represent strength and stability, a good representation for HEALTH. If you have your bathroom or a part of your bathroom in HEALTH of the house, you may want to hang a small chime on or above the door to the bathroom to negate the Water element aspect of the bathroom in your HEALTH area as, if you remember from Chapter 5, a chime stops Ch'i from continuing in a straight line so it will stop Ch'i from enhancing a negative situation. You may also want to use this same "cure" if a bathroom is located in the CAREER, WEALTH, FAME, or LOVE "life areas" of the structure.

In all cases and in all "life areas," you should always keep bathroom doors closed, toilet lids down, and shower curtains pulled closed to keep Ch'i from flowing out of your home or business.

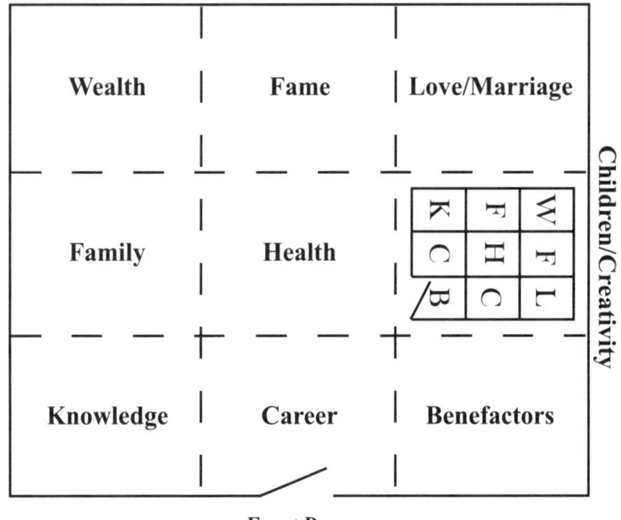

Chapter 19

House Ba-Gua vs. Room Ba-Gua

The "life areas" of a house are based on the front door entrance, symbolically the "mouth" which draws the "vital breath" (Ch'i) into the "lungs" of the house. The "life areas" of a room are based on the doorway into each room for "people flow" and "Ch'i flow."

First we do the Ba-gua of the house and then a Ba-gua for each room. As you can see from the diagram, this room is totally within CHILDREN/CREATIVITY of the house. Let's say this home is owned by an artist, and the room is the studio. When enhancing a room, remember enhancements should correspond to the "life area(s)" of the home, as the House Ba-gua takes precedence over any room Ba-gua. Now, lets enhance each "life area" of the studio.

In the CAREER area of the room I would place the desk which would contain such items as portfolios, the telephone, records of clients, the rolodex and a water fountain or water representation such as a small fish sculpture.

In the KNOWLEDGE area, I would recommend the storage shelves (metal shelves would be best as it is Creativity of the house and Creativity is ruled by Metal) for the paints and brushes be placed there and kept neat, clean and uncluttered.

In the FAMILY area (which includes "spiritual" family—people of like mind and goals), place any and all membership certificates and awards from any artists or professional associations to which they belong in *plastic frames* (plastic because FAMILY is ruled by wood but Creativity is ruled by metal).

In the WEALTH area, as it is in the Creativity area of the home, I would place a fountain to symbolize a constant flow of income from creative endeavors.

In the FAME area, place one of the artist's most noted works here, along with framed copies of newspaper articles, and awards. It will enhance their fame through their creative endeavors.

In the LOVE area, I would place the artwork with which they are the most satisfied. This will continue their love for their work. Add a picture of him/her with their significant other in a metal frame (the room is in the Creativity area of the house, whose element is metal). A metal-framed mirror will bring Ch'i into the room *and* enhance the LOVE area as it is in a direct line to the entrance.

The CHILDREN/CREATIVITY area of this room is powerful. It is what I call a "Double area" (Creativity of the room is contained in the Creativity area of the home). This is where the easel should be placed to stimulate creative flow.

The BENEFACTORS area is very important. As the only space available is the wall behind the door, I would recommend a large message board with the business cards of gallery owners, agents, business clients, and so forth.

In the HEALTH area, I would recommend a throw rug with earth tones and some yellows (yellow is the color for Health). Because of the use of paints in the room, which may not be "carpet friendly," you could hang an Austrian crystal and/or amber with yellow thread from a light fixture or ceiling fan in the center of the room.

In this example, the room was located entirely within the CHILDREN/CREATIVITY "life area" of the structure. However, this is usually not the case. More often than not, a room can be within two or more "life areas" of the structure.

In the example below, the room is within the CHILDREN/CREATIVITY and the BENEFACTORS "life areas" of the structure. As you can see, the Love/Marriage, Children/Creativity, and Benefactors "life areas" of the room are contained within the BENEFACTORS "life area" of the structure. The enhancements to these three room "life areas" would need to correspond to BENEFACTORS of the structure.

Be sure to take this into account when you are enhancing each room. Every room will have an exceptionally auspicious area. In the example below, you will note that although the room does not have a "Double" Creativity area, it does have a "Double" Benefactors area.

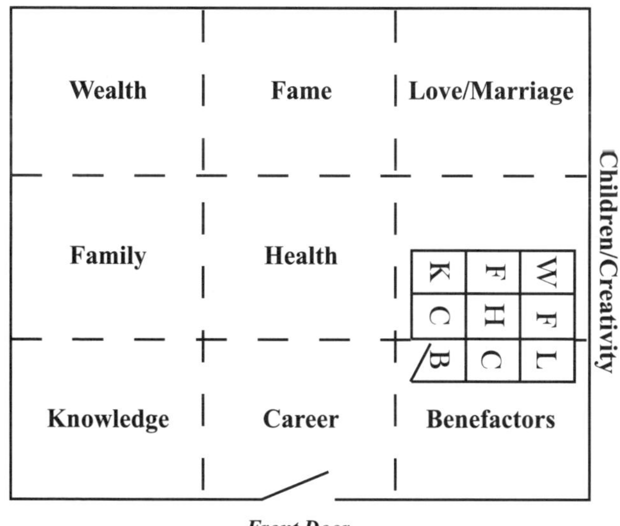

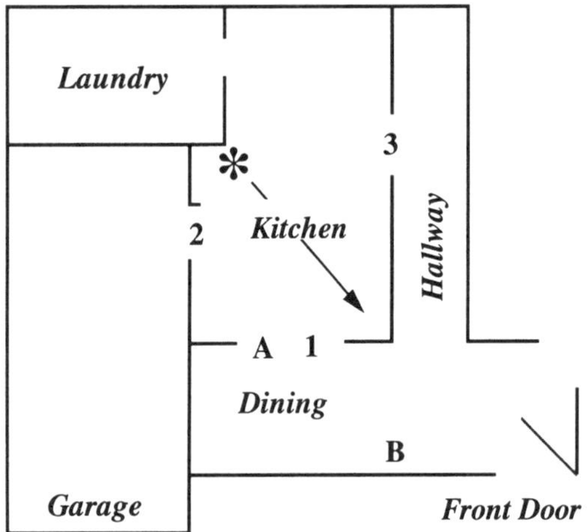

Chapter 20

Feng Shui Problem Solving

Multiple Entrances

In this chapter, we will look at the solution to the problem of correctly placing the Ba-Gua for a room which has more than one entrance. In our example we'll use the kitchen, as usually there are two or three entrances to get to the kitchen area in most homes.

Pictured is a diagram of the left 1/3 of a house. This side of the house has the garage, laundry room, kitchen, dining room, a hallway and the front door. As you can see, we have three ways to enter the kitchen. 1) is a wide entryway between the dining room and the kitchen, 2) is the entry to the kitchen from the garage and 3) is the entrance from the hallway. So, if we wanted to enhance the CAREER "life area" of the kitchen (remembering that the CAREER "life area" is the 1/3 central wall area where the entryway is), would the CAREER "life area" be at the Number 1, Number 2 or Number 3 entrance?

The first thing to remember in Feng Shui is that Ch'i (universal life force energy) translates literally as "vital breath" and that the front door entrance is the "mouth" which draws the Ch'i "vital breath" into the "lungs" of the house, so everything is based on the front door and, the only way Ch'i can enter a room is through the entrance to that room. We can eliminate Number 2, because we don't count the garage door as the front door entrance. Even if you use your garage door four times more often than the front door, it is still not considered the main entrance. The Ba-Gua for the garage would be based on how you enter it from the house, not by the garage door entrance.

The second thing to remember is that it is the nature of Ch'i to move in a straight line. Ch'i doesn't naturally make 90 degree angles (note that there are no 90 degree angles in nature). Therefore, you place the Ba-Gua of a room based on the least number of 90 degree angles that Ch'i has to make to enter a room from the front door. We can eliminate Number 3, because first the Ch'i heads straight into the wall across from the front door. Then it would have to make a 90 degree angle toward the Dining room. Then another 90 degree angle to go down the hall. And finally,

Ch'i would have to make another 90 degree angle to enter into the kitchen at Number 3.

It would be much easier for Ch'i to enter the kitchen at Number 1 by simply sweeping through the dining room from the front door. So, if we want to enhance this "life area" of the kitchen, now that we know where the CAREER "life area," and all of the other "life areas" are in the kitchen, all we have to do is place something there that has to do with the Element Water, the ear, and/or the color black. — But Wait!! We can't place anything there to enhance our career because all that's there is an open space!

Open Areas/Partial Walls

So, let's figure out how to "cure" open entrances to rooms (archway type entrances with no door), partial walls, and which "life areas" are affected by them.

Because of the large open entrance to the kitchen from the dining room, we actually have no CHILDREN/CREATIVITY "life area" in the dining room. This "life area" is just an open space. When we make another 90 degree turn to our right to be able to enter the kitchen from the dining room (turning the Ba-Gua with us), we see that the kitchen has no CAREER "life area" due to the same open entrance.

The best “cure” for this would be to place a small mirror where you see the Letter A in the diagram, which would “close off” the missing “life area” by reflecting the opposite wall. What we are doing, in effect, is creating a wall as, if you were invisible and looked into the mirror, all you would see is the opposite wall which is being reflected by the mirror. The mirror is “pulling in” the opposite wall to the wall it is on. This “closes” the missing area. Although we cannot place an enhancement in this area such as a water fountain or anything else because it would restrict the Ch’i flow of people being able to move freely between the rooms, at least we have the missing “life area” back.

I would also place a small mirror at the Letter B, as the entrance to the dining room is combined with the entrance foyer at the front door and the hallway. By reflecting the opposite wall, this would make the entrance to the dining room more defined, and give us back the entire BENEFACTORS, CAREER, and KNOWLEDGE “life areas” of the dining room.

A folding screen is also used in the Orient to “create a wall” but, in this case, I like the use of the mirrors better, as screens would restrict the free flow of movement.

You could probably think of several methods that have been used to create a wall or a door where there is an open entrance. Draperies which part in the middle have been used for centuries in the East and the West. Strung beads have been used in the East, and were popular in the West in the 60’s. In

Feng Shui, a shower curtain would "create a wall" between the bathtub and the rest of the bathroom.

Indoor Poison Arrows

Now we will look at what in Feng Shui is known as a "poison arrow", the effect it has on you and the "life areas" within your home or business, and how to "cure" it.

Look back once again at the diagram at the beginning of this chapter, and note the asterisk (*). A "poison arrow", is a protruding 90-degree angle which creates a sharp corner. Sharp corners cause Ch'i to flow too strongly in a direct line from the point of the corner. If we draw an imaginary line from the corner in a straight line out from the corner, anything in this pathway would be "weakened". "Poison arrows" also "weaken" any "life area" that they point at, and any "life area" they point through!

What we are seeking with Feng Shui is balance. Just like water, Ch'i that doesn't flow becomes "stagnant." Ch'i that flows too fast is like the raging water of a flood. What we are looking for is akin to a nice, meandering stream of energy. From the standpoint of energy flow, a sharp corner is like having a 100 lb per square inch fire hose that is turned on all the time and never runs out of water. The flow from this fire hose will "weaken" anything in its path, and anything it is directed at. I have demonstrated this in my classes, by muscle testing a student volunteer first, in the center of a room, and then again with the center of their back about 5 inches from a sharp corner. The volunteer is always surprised by the difference in their strength between the two tests.

As we had previously determined, the open entrance between the dining room and the kitchen is the correct entrance for determining where the "life areas" of the kitchen are located. We also see that the sharp corner is pointing at the BENEFACTORS "life area" of the kitchen which causes a "weakening" in our relationships with friends, helpful people and benefactors. Just as important is that the energy flow of the sharp corner passes through the center of the kitchen, which is the Health "life area" of the room and can cause a "weakening" of our physical well-being. This is especially significant as the kitchen is where we prepare our nutrition and abundance.

There are three "cures" to negate this problem. First is to place a potted plant (real or silk) in front of the corner or hang a plant with a trailing vine in such a way as the vine would be directly in front of the sharp corner to "soften" it. Second would be to hang an Austrian crystal (spherical) so that it is directly in front of the sharp corner. Third, is to use a mirror to extend the corner into a wall. This is the less preferable method, as by "creating a wall", it may change the Ba-Gua of a room.

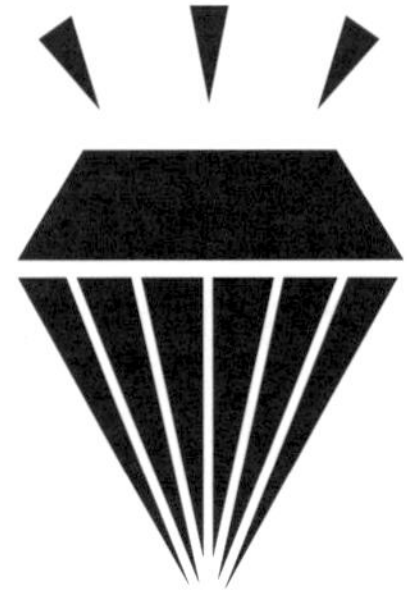

Chapter 21

Mineral Empowerment Feng Shui

After years of experimentation, I have found that placing one or more of the listed minerals, which are ranked from most powerful down, in their appropriate "life area" is a very powerful enhancement. I strongly encourage you to try them. You can place them on or in the soil of a potted or hanging plant, in a water fountain, on a mirror which will "double" their energy or on a quartz crystal cluster which will quadruple their energy.

It is important to note that the minerals listed in the LOVE/ RELATIONSHIP "life area" are to bring a ***NEW*** love into your life. If you wish to enhance and maintain a love relationship that you already have, place 1. Ruby*, 2. Red (Cherry) Amber, or 3. Rhyolite in this area.

The minerals listed in the FAME "life area" are to enhance how others see you. If you wish to see yourself in a better light or enhance your self-esteem, self-love or self-confidence, place 1. Rhodonite, 2. Rose Quartz*, 3. Hemomophite or 4. Carnelian in this area.

Do not combine stones which are "stimulators" and stones which are "soothers" as they can cancel each others energy out and have little to no effect. Minerals listed with an asterisk (*) after their names are considered "stimulators." For example, in the FAMILY "life area," do not place malachite (a stimulater) with turquoise (a soother). Try to place either all stimulators *or* all soothers in the same "life area." Using FAMILY as an example again, you would either place malachite and/or beryl there *or* you would place petrified wood, turquoise, jade, and/or shell in this "life area."

Avoid synthetic/man-made minerals. I have not experimented with all synthetics but all of the ones which I have tested do not have quite the same energy as natural minerals. In the case of minerals which can be very expensive, like emerald, ruby, and alexandrite, it would be better to go with small non-jewelry grade pieces rather than synthetics as the energy of natural minerals is the same regardless of grade or size.

WEALTH

1. Cinnabar* tie
1. Alexandrite*
2. Gold
3. Tektite
4. Ruby*
5. Chrysocolla*
6. Aventurine*

FAME

1. Carnelian
2. Bloodstone
3. Iron Pyrite
4. Fire Agate
5. Peridot*
6. Red Jade

LOVE - MARRIAGE

1. "Twin" Quartz Crystal*
2. Rhodochrosite
3. Moonstone
4. Pink/Rose Tourmaline*
5. Garnet*
6. Fire Opal

FAMILY

1. Petrified Wood
2. Malachite*
3. Turquoise
4. Beryl*
5. Jade
6. Shell

HEALTH

1. Amber tie
1. Nebula Stone
2. Bloodstone
3. Tiger's Eye
4. Bone/Ivory
5. Citrine/Smokey Quartz*
6. Dioptase*

CHILDREN

1. Silver
2. Rutilated Quartz (Silver Thread)*
3. Hematite*
4. Red Plume Agate
5. Moonstone
6. Pearl tie
6. Coral

KNOWL-EDGE

1. Amethyst*
2. Lapis*
3. Sodalite*
4. Emerald*
5. Turquoise
6. Opal

CAREER

1. Enhydro
2. Coral
3. Sea Shells
4. Aquamarine
5. Pearl
6. Adamite*

BENEFAC-TORS

1. Quartz Crystal Cluster*
2. Magnetite
3. Geode*
4. Tourmalated Quartz*
5. Desert Rose
6. Hyperstene

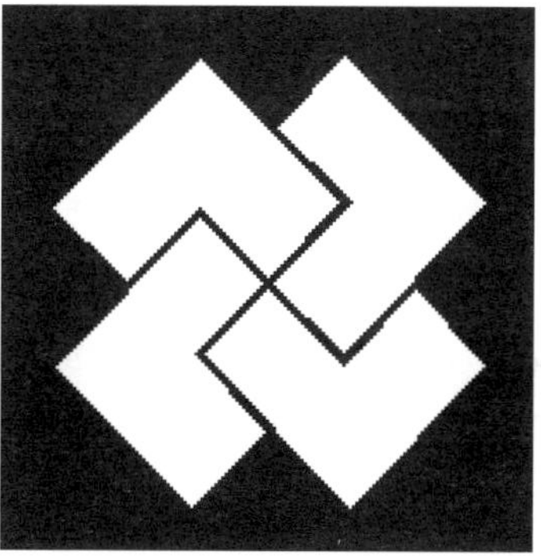

Chapter 22

Geometric Shapes in Feng Shui

I have found that it is very powerful Feng Shui to balance your home or business and/or a room within your home or business building structure using geometric shapes.

I based this method of Feng Shui on the "Color Wheel" that you probably remember from art class in school. One of my apprentices once showed me on her Color Wheel that any straight line or geometric shape drawn inside the Color Wheel will *always* touch "complimentary" colors. I decided to experiment with this using the Ba-Gua of Feng Shui and have found it to be most auspicious.

For example, if you place an enhancement in the WEALTH "life area" of a room, you should also place an enhancement in the LOVE "life area" to balance the room. It is also best to try to go with the same enhancement and the same number of enhancements in the "life areas." So, if you have two potted plants in the WEALTH "life area" of a room, there should be two plants in the LOVE "life area" of the same room. Otherwise there would be too much power or weight in just one corner of the room. If you have placed something powerful as an enhancement in the FAME "life area" of a room, there should be something equally powerful in the CAREER "life area" of the room (geometrically forming a straight line down the center of the room).

You could also form the shape of a triangle within a room by placing an enhancement in the FAME, KNOWLEDGE and BENEFACTORS "life areas" of a room. These are the three main "life areas" I like to enhance in a child or teenagers' room as KNOWLEDGE will help them in school, FAME will help them see themselves in a more powerful light, and BENEFACTORS will help them find mentors and teachers who will help them in their growth. Or, you could form a triangle within a room if we placed enhancements in the WEALTH, LOVE and CAREER "life areas."

Something interesting to note is the fact that I consider the KNOWLEDGE, FAME and BENEFACTORS triangle as the mental and spiritual reality and the WEALTH, LOVE and CA-

REER "life areas" as the material reality. The two triangles form the "Star of David" and is also considered the symbol of primal fire and primal water, others see the symbol of "as above, so below."

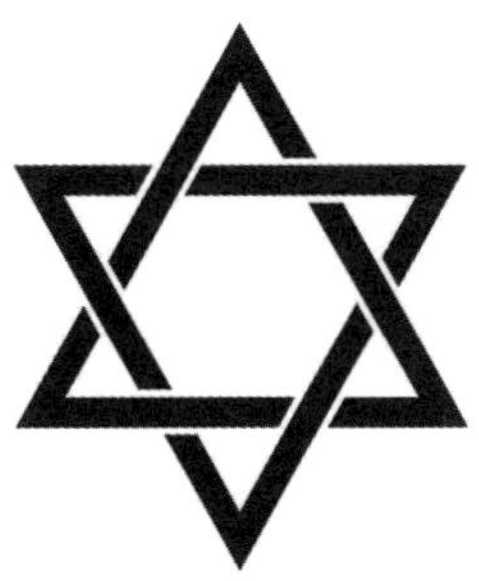

Whenever possible, it is very powerful to enhance the four corners of a room with the same enhancement and the same number of enhancements. For example, we could place a plant in the KNOWLEDGE, WEALTH, LOVE and BENEFACTORS areas forming a square within the square of the room (the square is a symbol of stability). Of course, if the door of a room opens in the KNOWLEDGE or BENEFACTORS "life area" of a room, this would not work as people trying to enter the room would either be hitting the planter pot (whether it were on the floor or hanging) with the door if it opens in or they would have to struggle to get around the plant if the door opens out.

As I have been using a room in these examples, remember to choose your enhancements in accordance with the Ba-Gua of the building structure as the building Ba-Gua takes precedence over the room Ba-Gua (see Chapter 19). If the room in the above example is in the CHILDREN/CREATIVITY "life area" of the home or building, we should not use plants as plants represent the Wood element and CHILDREN/CREATIVITY vibrates to the Metal element. Wood and Metal are considered conflicting elements (just like Water and Fire).

Generally, you are safe in enhancing the four corners of the building structure with the same element (a plant represents the Wood element, a rock represents the Earth element, etc.) as the four corners of the Ba-Gua do not have an element. The Chinese use a five element system and there are nine "life areas" of the Ba-Gua so not every "life area" has an element (see cover picture of the Ba-Gua). The "life areas" of the Ba-Gua that do vibrate to an element form a cross in the center of the Ba-Gua. CAREER is Water, FAMILY is Wood, FAME is Fire, HEALTH is Earth and CHILDREN/CREATIVITY is Metal.

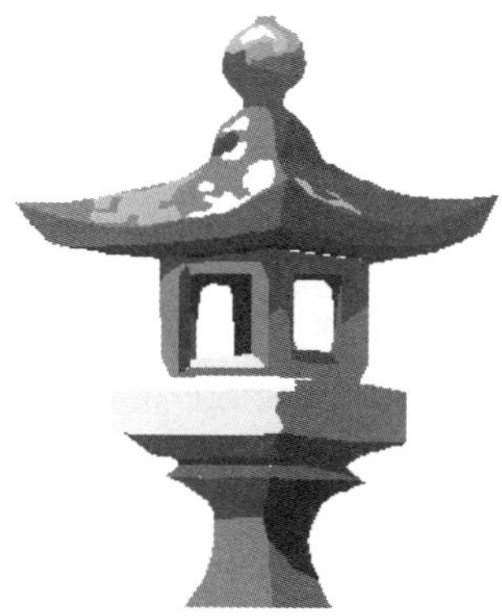

Chapter 23

Conscious Intent & Affirmations

Affirmations are not considered a traditional Feng Shui enhancement but they are very powerful and can change your life for the better.

First, according to Webster, an affirmation is something you "state emphatically." For an affirmation to work, you first have to state it - say it out loud. The throat is the area of manifestation. Sound is energy! What was "In the beginning" in Genesis? The Light? No - In the beginning was "**The Word**." Have you ever heard the saying "Be careful what you ask for - you might get it."? This saying isn't as negative as it sounds. It is just good advise to be positive and be specific in what you ask for. Since the beginning of time, our ancient ancestors have done this in the form of prayers or blessings. In this century, affirmations also became very popular in the business world as the main basis of PMA (Positive Mental Attitude).

Second, to state something "emphatically," you have to *believe* it. There has to be a conscious intent and it has to become your truth. When you say an affirmation, you can't be "wishy-washy" with the intent or the affirmation. If you want to attract love into your life, you can't say something like "Well, ah, even though my last relationship was a disaster, I think I'm kinda sorta ready for a new relationship." You would say something like "I am **now** ready to give and receive love!" There can be no half-intents. I had a client who wanted to use a room for entertaining but she did nothing in the room itself to make it be used for that purpose and did nothing to draw people to the room. It was like a room which was disconnected from the rest of the home. We turned the half-intent into a full intent by decorating the room appropriately for entertaining guests and used runner type carpets to draw people into the room.

Conscious intent is a major part of what makes Feng Shui work. When you, for instance, place a plant in your LOVE/RELATIONSHIP "life area," the physical action of doing this backed up with your conscious intent is like saying that you definitely want to make a positive change in this area of your life. When doing any enhancement, place your intent and the energy you want to manifest from the enhancement such as more passion in my marriage, better creative flow, etc.

Quantum physics proves that consciousness is the only true reality. You not only shape your own ideas through your conscious intent, you actually shape your physical reality through it. One of the best ways of proving this to yourself is to attend a Firewalk. I personally have attended Firewalks to "walk my talk" (no pun intended) and as a self-empowerment tool. If you can do that, you can do *anything*. To this day, our modern science cannot explain how people are able to walk across hot coals and not be burned. Being a "serious student" of martial arts for over 20 years, I have seen Masters of various styles of martial arts do things in demonstrations that modern science would say was physically impossible.

One of the best ways of making positive changes in your life is to use the power of your own conscious intent through affirmations. Write an affirmation on a piece of paper, believe it and say it out loud once with the full faith that it will happen. You only have to say it once with belief. (You don't have to say it 47 times a day and beat the Universe to death with it! You were heard the first time! If you called me 47 times a day, I'd quit answering the phone!) Roll up the piece of paper into a scroll, tie a red ribbon around it, and place it somewhere within the "life area" where you want to make a positive change. Make up your own affirmations, they are much more powerful. For instance, if you want a raise, use an affirmation like "I am recognized and rewarded for my work!" and place it in your CAREER "life area." If you want to increase your money flow, write something like "I attract money and abundance to myself each and every day!" and place it in your WEALTH "life area." In all the "life areas" but especially in the WEALTH "life area," I like to place the scrolled affirmation in an open basket, with the basket representing something ready to be filled. I recently had one of my Feng Shui students tell me that after trying to sell her house for over a year, she placed an affirmation to sell her home in a basket in her BENEFACTORS "life area" and her home sold four days later!

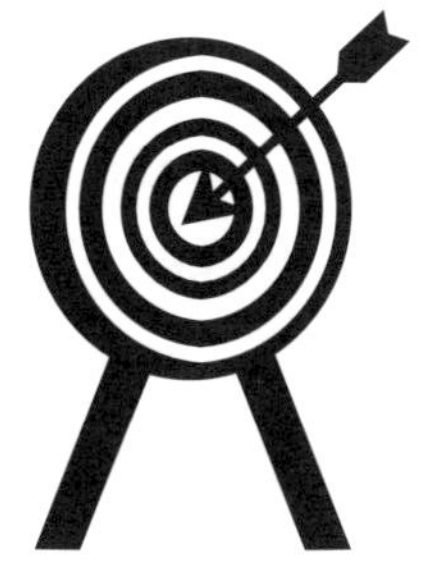

Chapter 24

Trouble Shooting

Now let's explore what to do if there is a stoppage or reversal following your enhancement of a "life area." As I mentioned previously, you can't totally avoid the universal law of what I call the "rising and falling," Feng Shui turns the peaks and valleys of life experience (sometimes called "feast or famine") into gently rolling hills. What we are looking at here is what to do if life suddenly starts going back to the extremes of peaks and valleys, after enhancing your environment.

Let's say you enhanced your CAREER & WEALTH "life areas" and immediately more business started flowing in, or you got a raise, and everything was really moving up for a few months. Then suddenly everything seemed to stop—the business flow started drying up, your car engine burned up, there is the sudden and untimely death of your refrigerator, etc.

In this situation, there are six questions I would ask. I have found one or more of the following are usually the reason(s) for the sudden change in nine out of ten cases.

1. *Did you consecrate your house?* This should be done before any enhancements. See Chapter 3.

2. *Did you neglect doing one or both of the two most important enhancements?* Placing a wind chime outside your front door to bring Ch'i to your front door area, and placing a mirror or hanging an Austrian crystal inside your home in a direct line to the center of the front door to bring the Ch'i in.

3. *Did you place a protective symbol in your home within sight of your front door to dispel negative Ch'i?* Any symbol that you have an affinity towards—an angel, a cross, a bear, tiger, lion, gargoyle, etc. (If you use an animal symbol, it should be ferocious looking—a cute stuffed toy tiger won't dispel anything.)

4. *Did you move anything, change anything, or place too many enhancements in a "life area?"* This is one of the top reasons for a sudden change in the flow of positive energy. I strongly believe in an old saying: "If it ain't broke—don't fix it!"

One client who, after experiencing major increases in her money flow, had a sudden reversal. I discovered that she had placed a small piece of amethyst in her WEALTH area. Any form of quartz puts out major energy and amethyst is a form of quartz, and the most powerful spiritual stone there is, which is a negative in the WEALTH area even though it is one of the colors (purple) of the area. Her money flow increased again immediately after I removed the amethyst from her WEALTH area and placed it in her KNOWLEDGE area!

Remember also the concept the Chinese call "FU", which is the concept of cyclic reversal. If anything in the universe goes too far to one extreme, the universe will take it to its exact opposite to create balance. So, if you changed things by adding "too much" to any "life area", the results will be the exact opposite of what you are trying to do. It's like using a 20 pound sledgehammer to crack open a walnut - all you get is nut dust.

5. *Did you enhance the "life areas" with representations of past failures?* Sometimes we are too focused on the enhancement itself, and not on its energy. One client enhanced the LOVE/RELATIONSHIP area of her living room with a beautiful vase, and her bedroom with an Austrian crystal in the shape of a heart. The problem was that the vase was a gift from her ex-husband, and the heart, which was a single heart and would represent a heart alone, was a gift from an ex-boyfriend.

<u>In every situation</u>, when you look at any enhancement, ask yourself three questions:

What does it mean to you?

Where did it come from?

What is the energy behind it?

Question number 6 relates to "life areas" which should be enhanced when, on the surface, you feel that the lack or limitations you are experiencing are in a "life area" which seems more obvious.

6. *Did you enhance the correct "life area" for the problem? Could there be deeper issues involved and/or do you have negative/self-destructive thoughts or mind-sets?*

For example, no matter how well you enhance your CAREER "life area," if you have a fear of success, things will go great, and then, when you get too close to reaching a certain point, you self-destruct. As mentioned in Chapter 12, if you enhance your WEALTH "life area" and the next day, while paying bills, you say out loud, "There is never enough!," you'll be right—there will never be enough. Or, if you believe that "Money is the root of all evil," you will always be broke, as no one wants anything "evil" around themselves.

If you enhanced your LOVE "life area" because you feel you can't maintain a good love relationship, but you have abandonment issues, you will always get caught up in that vicious cycle. You start a good relationship but your abandonment issues make you try to "grasp tighter." This causes the significant other to back away a few steps. You feel this backing away so you try to grasp even tighter, which causes the significant other to leave. This adds credence to your abandonment issues, and you try to grasp the next person even more tightly, and so forth.

In these examples, there is a need to change consciousness or intent. That is why, as I mentioned in Chapter 10, you always, always, *always* (did I say you should always?) enhance your KNOWLEDGE/SELF-KNOWLEDGE "life area." By enhancing this area, you will learn what you need to build on and what to release in order to grow.

In the last example, you saw that the "life area" which needed to be enhanced was KNOWLEDGE/SELF-KNOWLEDGE, when enhancing LOVE would have been more obvious on the surface. Another good example of this would be the situation of a client who felt she needed more powerful enhancements in her WEALTH "life area." I recommended we should first do more in the "life area" which is diagonally across from WEALTH, the BENEFACTORS area. This was the correct area to enhance. As she felt that "the only way to get the job done right is to do it yourself," she was restricting WEALTH by disallowing BENEFACTORS/HELPFUL PEOPLE to come into her life. This made the difference in her personal and business situation.

In all cases, you should enhance every "life area" of the Ba-Gua. In some, you may need to take a closer look at a "life area" which is directly or diagonally across from the area where you feel lack or limitation.

Ending Note to the Reader

This should give you enough basic information to get your Ch'i flowing and make a positive impact on your life.

Again, before you do any enhancements, it is best to read the entire book first to absorb the concepts. Start out slowly with your enhancements.

First, consecrate your home or business (see Chapter 3). "Square off" your structure (see Chapter 7), if needed. Then, place a chime in a direct line to the center of the front door or above the center of the front door. Finally, place a mirror or austrian crystal inside your structure in a direct line to the center of the front door.

Go about four weeks and see how the shift in energy feels. Keep a journal during this period to record any changes you notice or that others notice.

Add ***one*** enhancement to each "life area" in the house or a room every two to four weeks. This is the only way you will be able to see which enhancements are working for you. If, for example, you place an enhancement in the LOVE "life area" of three rooms in your structure and you only notice a slight difference in the energy and in your love life; you won't know which one of the three is helping and which two are doing nothing or may be actually detracting from the LOVE energy.

I cannot over emphasize how powerful the use of

minerals is in Feng Shui. I have spent years of research, first experimenting with mineral placements in "life areas" in my own home to test the effect of the mineral's energy, then trying it with other people I was doing consultations with. All minerals have a unique energy but I have only listed ones which I have tested and I know work.

In all cases, trust your intuition in how each enhancement feels to you. Remember that no matter what you read in any book, if you are going to throw negative energy at any recommended enhancement or "cure" because it doesn't feel right to you, try to find a *creative* way to use the enhancement/ "cure" that you can live with. If you can't... *don't use it*! Go with a creative alternative which fits you and your decor.

The most important thing is balance. You don't want to, for instance, go against a Universal Law, but you also do not want to get bogged down with over-analyzing details. **Just trust what you feel and have fun with it.**

Bibliography

A Book Of Five Rings - Miyamoto Musashi, Translated by Victor Harris, The Overlook Press, 1974.
A Soul In Place, Reclaiming Home as Sacred Space, Carol Bridges, Earth Nation Publishing, 1995.
Chinese Symbolism And Art Motifs, C.A.S. Williams, Charles E. Tuttle Company, Inc., 1974.
Edgar Cayce On The Power Of Color, Stones, And Crystals, Dan Campbell, Warner Books, Inc., 1989.
Feng Shui - A Layman's Guide to Chinese Geomancy, Evelyn Lip, Times Editions PTE LTD, 1979, American edition - Heian International, Inc., 1987.
Feng Shui for The Home, Evelyn Lip, Times Editions PTE LTD, 1986, American edition - Heian International, Inc., 1990.
Feng Shui The Chinese Art of Placement, Sarah Rossbach, Penguin Group/Arkana, 1991.
Interior Design with Feng Shui, Sarah Rossbach, Penguin Group/Arkana, 1991.
Lao-tzu's Tao Te Ching, Translated by Red Pine, Mercury House, 1996.
Lao Tzu's Tao Te Ching, Translated by Thomas H. Miles, Avery Publishing Group Inc., 1992.
Love Is In The Earth - A Kaleidoscope Of Crystals, Melody, Earth-Love Publishing House, 1991.
Stone Power, Dorothee L. Mella, Warner Books, Inc., 1988.

Index

About The Author

Phoenix (aka David Nutter, aka Steve Tomblyn) is a Feng Shui Master, Reiki Master, T'ai Chi Instructor, and has two Black Belts in Karate. He has studied the energy of minerals and the healing system of Reiki for over 10 years, Taoism and Feng Shui for over 15 years, and has studied Martial Arts and the power of Ch'i for over 20 years.

He started studying religions, philosophies, ancient cultures, spirituality, metaphysics, and mind expansion at the age of 14 and adeptly integrates and draws on his comprehensive knowledge of these subjects in his writing and teaching.

As a writer and teacher, he has the unique ability to make even the most complex concepts easy, understandable, and fun.

He is available for workshops, classes, seminars, and speaking engagements and is accepting apprentices in the Art and Science of Feng Shui.

In addition to Feng Shui, he also teaches classes in Reiki, T'ai Chi, Karate, Self-defense, Women's and Men's Self-Empowerment, Taoism, Crystal Awareness, Crystal Healing, and Prosperity.

You can contact him through the publisher at:

Phoenix
c/o Perfect Harmony, Inc.
2533 N. Carson St. Box P316
Carson City, NV. 89706

Ba-Gua in a Square Layout

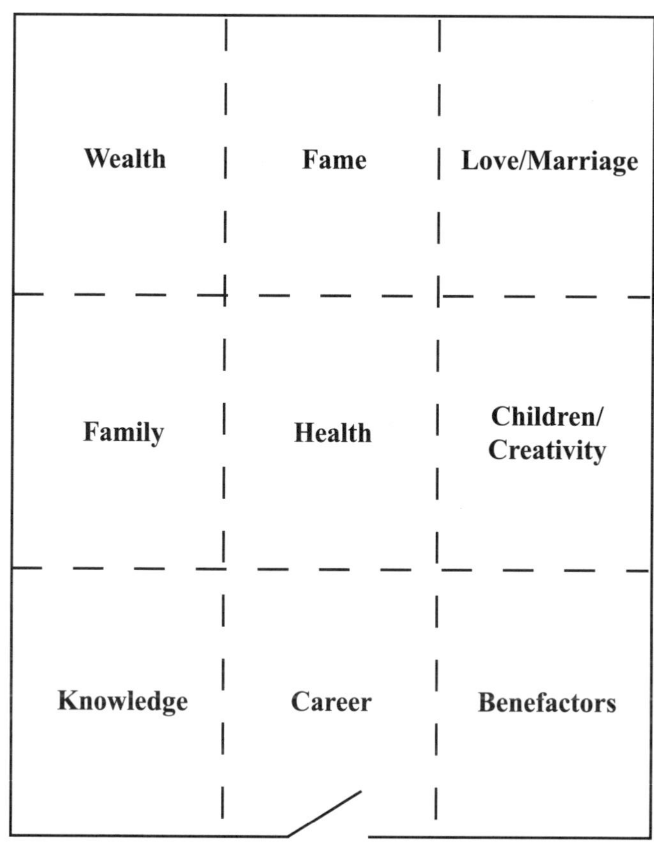

See traditional Ba-Gua on next Page.

Traditional Ba-Gua

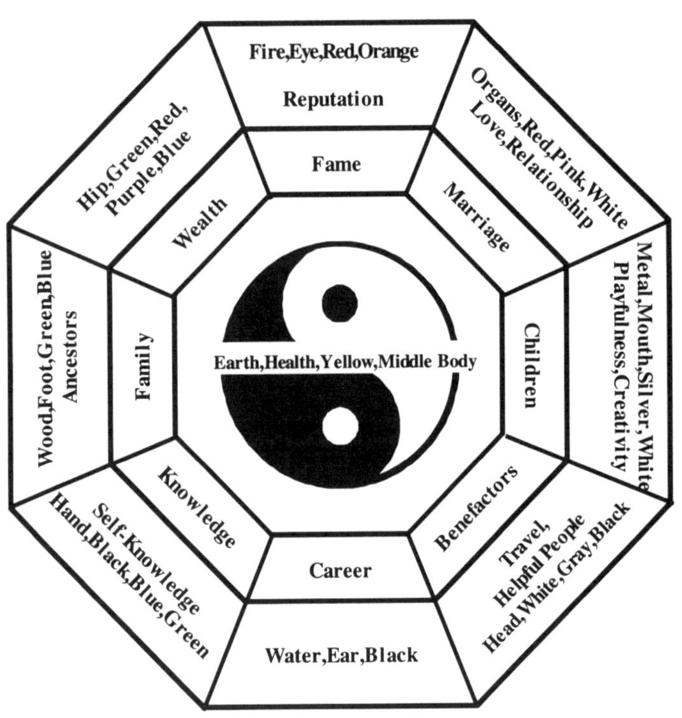

TESTIMONIALS

"After taking a Feng Shui course from David Nutter, I was able to bring balance and harmony into my life which manifested itself in two major ways:

Just six weeks into a new job, I was unexpectedly given a $3,000 annual salary increase.

I now have an overall sense of feeling better about myself which resulted in a higher level of self-esteem. This change in my mind set affects all other areas of my life.

Having the Feng Shui concept in my life makes so much sense to me......"

GLM, Morgantown, WV

"After you did the Feng Shui consultation for me on my home, I am feeling much more content and spiritually satisfied. My emotions and mood are happier and I definitely have a more positive outlook on life.

The mineral you recommended to place in my two childrens rooms have caused a tremendous change in their behavior. They get along much better, their attitudes have become positive, and their grades have improved!"

Linda S., Fairmont, WV

"The most significant change I've seen is that the peaks and valleys of my life have been replaced by gently rolling hills of experience!"

MDH, Albuquerque, NM

"The last company I worked for went out of business and I desperately searched for work for over 9 months. Then David Nutter did a reading on my house, made adjustments in my Career, Fame, and Benefactors areas and two weeks later I found a wonderful job.

Dave Nutter is the greatest!"

P. Ward, Albuquerque, NM

"I had had a Feng Shui consultation on my home by a consultant from a different school of Feng Shui. One year later, Dave went through my house and I saw immediate improvement in various areas of my life.

At first I was nervous that my house would look like a Chinese restaurant and was surprised that the "treatments" blended so well with my decor that they were barely detectable.

Within weeks, I received a $4,500 insurance reimbursement which, after waiting two years, I had given up on. Addi-

tionally, men started crawling out of the woodwork. I found this turn of events very interesting and quite delightful.

I have more direction and focus. Tremendous opportunities continue to emerge and life has once again become an incredible adventure.

HT, Pagosa Springs, CO

After experiencing profound results in my home, I filled my sons hand with some minerals Dave recommended to me the first opportunity I had to visit my son who lives in another state.

Within ten days, he landed the job he had wanted for months and went from homeless to an apartment of his own.

If you are looking for quick and definite results, I highly recommend Dave's suggestions on the power of minerals.

BSM, Tacoma, WA

I met Dave in the Spring of 1996. At the time, I was finding it very difficult to recover from the loss of my husband 3 1/2 years earlier and I was shifting between bouts of depression and loneliness and earnest efforts to restore my interest in life. I decided to ask Dave for a Feng Shui consultation.

Dave walked through my home explaining the "life areas" and identified those that needed addressing. He expressed concern that in addition to my LOVE area, the KNOWLEDGE area was very weak. I was somewhat startled as I had been struggling with identifying what my purpose was in life and always coming up empty.

Around two months later, I met my David. We were married in the Fall of 1997. I believe the Feng Shui helped me in all areas of my life.

DS, Rio Rancho, NM

I honestly and truly believe that I wouldn't have been able to buy my home without Feng Shui. I got a promotion from manager to director with a substantial raise (9.5% and the norm is 3 to 4%).

Feng Shui has really worked for me!

AB, El Paso, TX

David is blessed with an amazing gift. He truly understands the art of Feng Shui.

After he showed us how to make adjustments in our home, we saw an incredible growth in our career and income - we have more than doubled our salary!

GG and JJ, Albuquerque, NM